A Laboratory Course in
TISSUE
ENGINEERING

Melissa Kurtis Micou
and Dawn M. Kilkenny

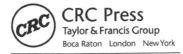
CRC Press
Taylor & Francis Group
Boca Raton   London   New York

CRC Press is an imprint of the
Taylor & Francis Group, an **informa** business

CRC Press
Taylor & Francis Group
6000 Broken Sound Parkway NW, Suite 300
Boca Raton, FL 33487-2742

Version Date: 20120713

International Standard Book Number: 978-1-4398-7893-4 (Paperback)

Library of Congress Cataloging-in-Publication Data

Micou, Melissa Kurtis.
   A laboratory course in tissue engineering / Melissa Kurtis Micou and Dawn M. Kilkenny.
     p. ; cm.
   Includes bibliographical references and index.
   ISBN 978-1-4398-7893-4
   I. Kilkenny, Dawn M. II. Title.
   [DNLM: 1. Tissue Engineering--methods--Laboratory Manuals. QT 25]

610.28--dc23
                                                  2012007453

Visit the Taylor & Francis Web site at
http://www.taylorandfrancis.com

and the CRC Press Web site at
http://www.crcpress.com

Contents

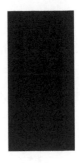

Chapter 10. Cell Patterning Using Microcontact Printing 109

Chapter 11. Measuring and Modeling the Motility of a Cell
                 Population Using an Under-Agarose Assay 121

Chapter 14.   Effect of Culture Configuration (Two versus Three Dimensions) on Matrix Accumulation 161

Chapter 15.   Combining In Silico and In Vitro Techniques to Engineer Pluripotent Stem Cell Fate............................ 173

Preface

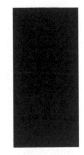

During the past decade, there has been a tremendous increase in the number of engineering programs offering undergraduate lecture courses in tissue engineering. The benefits of hands-on experience in this applied and interdisciplinary field are evident, yet very few programs offer associated lab courses. The small number of existing tissue-engineering lab courses may be attributed, in part, to the lack of available instructional materials. Preparation of this textbook was prompted by the numerous requests the authors and contributors received for the protocols used in their courses and the hope that more lab courses in tissue engineering will be offered to students in the near future. In particular, the book contains experiments suitable for (1) upper division undergraduate students with knowledge of engineering fundamentals, cell biology, and statistics or (2) graduate students who are new to the field.

The experiments within this book are based on both classic tissue-engineering experiments and recent advances in the field. The exercises in Chapter 3 and experiments in the early chapters help students master the techniques necessary to complete the more sophisticated experiments contained in later chapters. This collection of experiments was assembled to encompass a set of widely applicable techniques: cell culture, microscopy, histology, immunohistochemistry, mechanical testing, soft lithography, and common biochemical assays. In addition to teaching these specific techniques, the experiments emphasize engineering analysis, mathematical modeling, and statistical experimental design.

The content and structure of the book are intended to facilitate development of new tissue-engineering lab courses. Fifteen stand-alone experiments provide significantly more than a semester's worth of activities, allowing instructors to customize their courses. Most experiments conform to a schedule commonly used in undergraduate lab courses (i.e., 2- to 4-hour sessions once or twice a week). For added flexibility, experiments are broken up into as many different sessions as possible. The textbook provides students with a list of available materials that they will find in the lab for each experiment. Additional information, including suppliers and product numbers, is available in the instructor's manual along with other resources to help plan a new course.

The investment required to establish an instructional tissue-engineering lab facility can be substantial; therefore, the experiments make extensive use of a shared set of equipment, summarized in Table 1.1 in Chapter 1. Due to the interdisciplinary nature of tissue engineering, it is possible to use this shared set of equipment to conduct experiments that reinforce a wide range of engineering and life science concepts covered in typical biomedical engineering and bioengineering programs.

It is important for engineering students to develop strong communication skills to document and disseminate their work. The data analysis and reporting section within each chapter provides a framework for succinctly documenting the key results from each experiment. Additionally, Chapter 19 provides guidelines for reporting results in the form of a technical report or journal article, extended abstract, abstract, or technical poster. In our experience, varying the specific report format exposes students to common modes of scientific communication and is also more enjoyable for the students.

We hope that you find the experiments in this textbook representative of the exciting and dynamic field of tissue engineering.

Melissa Kurtis Micou, PhD
University of California, San Diego

Dawn M. Kilkenny, PhD
University of Toronto

Acknowledgments

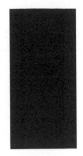

I am grateful for the contributions of my colleagues in the Department of Bioengineering at the University of California, San Diego (see contributors section). In particular, I would like to thank Dr. Robert Sah for introducing me to the field of tissue engineering years ago and for inspiring several experiments contained within this textbook. I also thank Doug Gurevitch for overseeing operation of the bioengineering instructional lab. I appreciate the efforts of the students, teaching assistants, and friends who helped refine these experiments and proofread the text, especially Mark Chapman, Todd Johnson, Kelvin Li, Joyce Luke, Hermes Taylor-Weiner, Justin Tse, Chris Villongco, and Ludovic Vincent. I would like to recognize the Tissue Engineering and Regenerative Medicine International Society (TERMIS) and Kristen Billiar, in particular, for organizing a session on undergraduate education at the 2010 EU meeting. The session served as the catalyst for this book by introducing me to the ambitious work of my coauthor and her colleagues at the University of Toronto. On a personal note, I thank my husband, Paul, for his constant support.

—Melissa Kurtis Micou

My involvement with this textbook stems from my association with the Institute of Biomaterials and Biomedical Engineering (IBBME) undergraduate teaching laboratory at the University of Toronto. In the few years I have been associated with this facility, the enthusiasm of the undergraduate students and the dedication of the graduate student teaching assistants has reiterated the importance of establishing a "protocol network," which we are able to do with this book. I am extremely grateful for the contributions of my colleagues at the IBBME (see contributors section). I would also like to thank Dr. Jonathan Rocheleau (IBBME) for editing and countless helpful discussions, as well as Laura Izakelian for time invested in testing various cell adhesion culture conditions. Similarly, I truly appreciate the full support given to this textbook by both Dr. Peter Zandstra (IBBME) and Dr. Craig Simmons (IBBME). Special thanks to my coauthor Dr. Melissa Kurtis Micou for inviting me to participate in the creation of this exciting book! Finally, my contributions would not have been possible without the support of my husband, Jon, and my children, Ben, Liam, Madeleine, Andrew, and Ian.

—**Dawn M. Kilkenny**

Authors

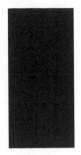

Melissa Kurtis Micou, PhD, is a lecturer in the Department of Bioengineering at the University of California, San Diego. She has taught tissue-engineering lecture and lab courses for undergraduate students for the past 9 years.

Dawn M. Kilkenny earned a PhD in physiology from the University of Western Ontario, Canada. Following postdoctoral studies in the field of growth factor research at Vanderbilt University, Nashville, Tennessee, she became a senior research specialist at the Vanderbilt Cell Imaging Shared Resource (CISR) microscope facility. Dr. Kilkenny is currently an assistant professor at the Institute of Biomaterials and Biomedical Engineering (IBBME), University of Toronto, and is academic advisor to the IBBME undergraduate teaching laboratory. Her research interests include cellular signaling, fluorescent protein technology, and microscopy.

Contributors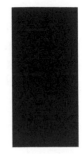

We greatly appreciate the contributions of many colleagues to the chapters included in this text. In particular, we extend thanks to the following for their specific contributions:

Paul Micou created the majority of illustrations, including all of those in Chapters 4–7 and 9–14.

Department of Bioengineering, University of California, Los Angeles:
Wujing Xian generously provided text and illustrations included in Chapters 1 and 3.

Institute of Biomaterials and Biomedical Engineering, University of Toronto:
Julie Audet generously contributed the protocol described in Chapter 15.

Geoff Clarke provided modeling software updates and user instructions for Chapter 15.

Jeffery Hoover provided valuable feedback, editing, and relevant questions for Chapter 18.

Whitaik David Lee provided valuable feedback for development of Chapter 15.

Jennifer Ma provided valuable feedback for development of Chapter 15.

Aaron Y. K. Ming provided feedback and created illustrations for Chapters 1, 3, 8, 15–18, and Appendix 5.

Faisal Moledina created the computational model described in Chapter 15.

Christopher Moraes generously contributed the protocol described in Chapter 17.

Mario Moscovici assisted with initial optimization of the protocol described in Chapter 15.

Kento Onishi created the computational model described in Chapter 15.

Lewis A. Reis provided valuable feedback and editing for Chapter 15.

Catherine Sammut assisted with creation of the protocol described in Chapter 15.

Craig A. Simmons generously provided the protocols and significant feedback regarding development of Chapters 16–18, as well as full support of this project from the onset.

Suthan Srigunapalan provided feedback, editing, and relevant questions for Chapter 16.

Edmond W. K. Young generously provided the protocol described in Chapter 16.

Peter W. Zandstra generously contributed the protocol described in Chapter 15 and provided full support of this project from the onset.

Department of Bioengineering, University of California, San Diego:

Karen Christman provided the protocol and feedback for development of Chapter 7.

Adam Engler provided the protocol and feedback for development of Chapter 13.

Noah Goshi assisted in protocol development and provided text and questions for Chapters 10 and 11.

Chapter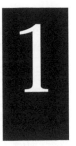

Getting Started in the Lab

1.1 Introduction

Tissue engineering is defined as the application of the principles and methods of engineering and the life sciences toward the fundamental understanding of structure–function relationships in normal and pathological mammalian tissue, as well as the development of biological substitutes to restore, maintain, or improve tissue function (Skalak and Fox 1988). Understanding structure–function relationships *and* developing biological substitutes are two distinct and important components of tissue engineering. The collection of experiments in this lab manual encompasses both of these areas.

Tissue engineering is a diverse and interdisciplinary field that involves the combined use of cells, biomaterials, chemical factors, and engineering methodologies. Conducting experiments successfully and safely in this field requires knowledge and preparation. To help orient you to the lab setting, this chapter describes equipment, supplies, and consumable reagents commonly found in a tissue-engineering lab.

1.2 A Well-Stocked Lab

Certain equipment, reagents, and disposable items are necessary for routine tissue-engineering lab work and are utilized extensively in the experiments contained within this book. Rather than repeatedly listing these items within individual chapters, Table 1.1 summarizes the general equipment and supplies found in a well-stocked tissue-engineering lab. It is assumed, throughout this text, that these materials are available. All the equipment, supplies, and consumables from this list are described in more detail in the following sections.

TABLE 1.1

General-Purpose Equipment, Supplies, and Consumables Needed for Experiments Contained in This Book

Equipment and Supplies	Consumables
Balance	Serological pipettes[a]
Glassware: beakers,[a] Erlenmeyer flasks, graduated cylinders, volumetric flasks, and bottles[a]	Pasteur pipettes[a]
	Pipette tips[a]
Small instruments: forceps,[a] scalpel handles,[a] and spatulas[a]	Weigh boats/weigh paper
Vortex mixer	Tissue culture vessels: petri dishes,[a]
Magnetic stir plate with stir bars[a]	flasks,[a] multiwell plates[a]
Orbital shaker	Conical centrifuge tubes[a]
Water purification system	Microcentrifuge tubes[a] and vials[a]
Pipette aids	Autoclave supplies
Micropipettes	Filters for liquid sterilization[a]
pH Meter	Syringes[a] and needles[a]
Centrifuge	Scalpel blades[a]
Refrigerator (4°C)	
–20°C freezer	
–80°C freezer and/or liquid nitrogen storage	
Biosafety cabinet (BSC)	
Vacuum pump or house vacuum (for liquid aspiration)	
CO_2 incubator	
Autoclave	
Inverted microscope with image capture	
Hemacytometer	

[a] A sterile supply of these items should be readily available.

1.3 Commonly Used Lab Equipment

- **Balance.** Top-loading electronic balances are commonly found in the lab and are categorized as either regular or analytical, depending on their capacity and weighing resolution or "readability." A regular balance has a capacity of hundreds to thousands of grams and readability from milligrams to grams. An analytical balance has a capacity of tens to hundreds of grams with a readability ≤ 0.1 mg. When weighing samples, choose the correct balance based on the weight of the sample and the precision required.

- **Glassware.** Beakers, Erlenmeyer flasks, graduated cylinders, volumetric flasks, and bottles of different sizes are examples of typical glassware used in a tissue-engineering lab. To clean glassware, first wash with detergent until free of residue (water will flow as a sheet rather than streaks on a clean glass surface); then rinse with tap water followed by deionized water (dH_2O).

- **Small instruments.** A supply of reusable forceps, scalpel handles, and spatulas for handling delicate samples, dissecting tissue, weighing reagents, and other routine tasks should be available at all times.

- **Mixing.** The vortex mixer, magnetic stirring plate, and orbital shaker are all examples of commonly used mixing equipment. There may also be requirements for specialized mixing equipment such as a sonicator or homogenizer, depending upon sample preparation requirements.

- **Vortex mixer.** The high-speed motion of a vortex mixer generates a vortex resulting in quick mixing of liquid–liquid or liquid–solid. It is generally used for quick mixing in containers such as microcentrifuge tubes or test tubes where vortexes can be readily generated.

- **Magnetic stir plate and stir bar.** This stirring platform is generally used for mixing liquids in beakers, flasks, bottles, or other larger containers. For efficient stirring, the length of a magnetic stirring bar should be approximately two-thirds the diameter of the container's base.

- **Orbital shaker.** This type of mixer is suitable for consistent mixing over a prolonged period of time. Some shakers are equipped with environmental control, such as a water bath that can maintain constant temperatures while shaking takes place. Conversely, a shaker can be placed into a temperature-controlled environment (such as a cold room or 4°C cooler) if required.

- **Water purification system.** Requirement of water purity depends upon the application. Water purity is categorized as types I, II, and III, corresponding to resistivities of >18.2 MΩ·cm, >1 MΩ·cm, and >50 kΩ·cm, respectively. For general reagent preparation, type I water is usually preferred. However, for less demanding use, such as glassware rinsing, type III water is usually sufficient. *Note that dH₂O water can be corrosive to metal; therefore, it may not be suitable for certain applications.* Deionization is achieved by filtering water through mixed-bed ion-exchange resins that remove both the anions and cations.

- **Equipment for liquid transfer.** Liquid transfer is handled in a manner dependent on the volume of liquid, liquid viscosity, and required accuracy. Micropipettes, electronic pipette aids, and transfer pipettes are some of the most commonly used liquid transfer tools.

  - **Pipette aids** are used with serological pipettes to handle moderate liquid volumes (generally, ~0.2–100 mL). Both the nosepiece of the pipette aid and the filter inside can be sterilized and are therefore appropriate for use in cell culture.

  - **Micropipettes** are more accurate for smaller liquid volumes (1 μL–1 mL) and are fully or partially sterilizable. As a consequence, these instruments are routinely used during cell culture protocols.

  - **Transfer pipettes** are used to transfer small volumes (<10 mL) from one container to another when accuracy is not required.

- **pH Meter.** This instrument is used for measuring the pH of solutions. Always read the instrument's operation manual before use. It is extremely important that the meter be calibrated on a regular basis using standard pH buffers. Likewise, the electrode should be stored in the proper storage buffer and never be allowed to dry out. *Never store the electrode in water* as it will cause ions to leach out of the glass bulb, making the electrode useless. However, dH₂O may be used to rinse the electrode each time it is moved to a new solution.

- **Centrifuges.** A variety of centrifuges are available depending upon the centrifugal force required for sample sedimentation. Typically, minicentrifuges and microcentrifuges are used for quick processing of small sample volumes (<2 mL each), whereas bench-top and floor model centrifuges accommodate larger volumes and offer more centrifugal power. For example, cells in suspension can be "collected" as a pellet by centrifugation at low speeds (i.e., <1000 g). Once the supernatant has been removed, the cells can be resuspended in fresh medium or buffer. This procedure is used to concentrate a cell sample or wash off a reagent.

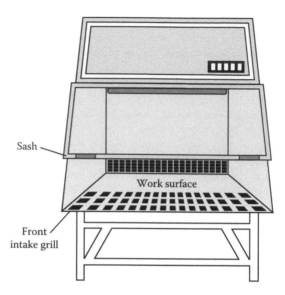

Sash

Work surface

Front
intake grill

Figure 1.1
Schematic of a typical class II BSC. The sterile environment and work surface within the BSC are maintained by the glass sash and curtain of HEPA-filtered air flowing to the front intake grill.

- **Refrigeration and frozen storage.** Some reagents require storage at temperatures below room temperature (4°C, −20°C, or −80°C). For any given reagent, refer to the label, product specification sheet, and/or material safety data sheet (MSDS) to determine the appropriate storage temperature. Typically, 4°C refrigeration is adequate for short-term storage of thawed reagents, whereas −20°C and −80°C freezers are used for long-term storage. In particular, it is important to minimize the number of freeze–thaw cycles when handling labile reagents such as enzymes and serum. It is also important to determine whether a frozen reagent should be thawed slowly on ice when removed from storage, or whether it may be quick-thawed in a warm water bath.

- **Liquid nitrogen storage and cryostorage.** This type of cold storage is generally in the form of a vacuum-insulated tank partly filled with liquid nitrogen. Cryostorage is typically used for long-term storage of frozen cells. The extremely low temperature of liquid nitrogen (−196°C) is crucial for maintaining cell viability. For safety reasons, frozen cells should be stored "dry" in the vapor phase of the liquid nitrogen and not fully submerged.

- **Class II biosafety cabinet (BSC).** A class II biosafety (or biological safety) cabinet is a contained workspace that provides a sterile environment for handling cells, tissue, and other biological samples (Figure 1.1). This type of workspace also provides protection for the worker from the potential hazards of the sample. Class I BSCs protect the environment and personnel but do not provide a sterile environment within the cabinet. Class III BSCs are necessary only for working with high-risk biological agents. All BSCs use high-efficiency particulate air (HEPA) filters to remove airborne particulates and aerosols larger than 0.3 μm, thus eliminating most airborne microbes. The filtered air is effectively sterile. BSCs are also generally equipped with germicidal UV lamps that eliminate potential microbial contamination when not in use (the UV lamp must be turned off when the BSC is in use). BSCs are commonly

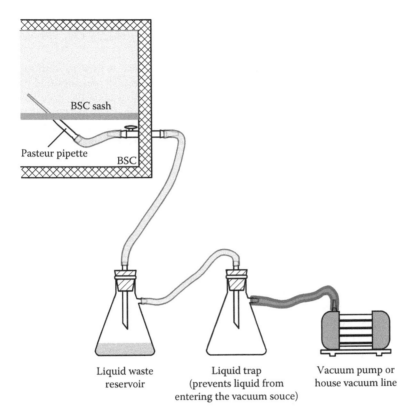

Figure 1.2
Use of a reservoir and liquid trap attached to a vacuum source allows liquid aspiration from samples within the sterile environment of the cabinet. (From Xian, W. 2009. *A Laboratory Course in Biomaterials.* Boca Raton, FL: CRC Press/Taylor & Francis. With permission.)

referred to as "hoods"; however, their function is vastly different from that of a chemical fume hood.

- **Vacuum pump or house vacuum for liquid aspiration.** There is often need to aspirate liquid from a sample (e.g., supernatant from a centrifuged cell suspension). A vacuum pump or house vacuum is sequentially connected to a liquid trap and waste reservoir (e.g., a vacuum flask) to establish an aspiration system. Sterile, disposable glass Pasteur pipettes can be attached to the vacuum inlet via appropriately sized tubing. As vacuum is applied, liquid is aspirated into the waste reservoir, where it is decontaminated with bleach. This accessory is typically found within a BSC for efficient liquid removal from cell culture flasks (Figure 1.2).

- **CO_2 incubator.** A CO_2 incubator provides a controlled environment for cell cultures, including a precise temperature, CO_2 level, high relative humidity, and HEPA-filtered air circulation to remove particulates. The CO_2 provided by the incubator works in conjunction with buffers present in tissue culture media to maintain a neutral pH. For this reason, it is important not to have cultures out of the incubator for extended periods of time. A typical CO_2 incubator is equipped with a thermostat and is water-jacketed to provide even heat distribution. The interior is usually constructed of stainless steel to prevent corrosion and to allow proper disinfection. The cell cultures used within this textbook can be maintained in standard incubator conditions (5% CO_2, 95% humidity, and an internal temperature of 37°C).

- **Autoclave (pressurized steam sterilizer).** An autoclave is used to sterilize equipment and reagents with high temperatures (≥120°C) and high pressures (≥15 psi). The actual temperature and duration settings vary depending upon the materials being autoclaved. Autoclaving can be used to sterilize glassware, small instruments, or large liquid volumes (e.g., multiple 1 L bottles at one time). Not all components can withstand the high temperatures associated with autoclaving. For instance, PBS contains inorganic salts and can be autoclaved, while culture media contain organic compounds that are inactivated at high temperatures. It is important to note that autoclaving of liquid requires slow exhaustion of steam.

- **Water bath.** A water bath maintained at 37°C is necessary for thawing and prewarming reagents and cells to physiological temperature. The bath water should be changed periodically to prevent microbial overgrowth. *Important: bottles, tubes, and other containers should not be fully submerged in a water bath as the contained reagents risk being contaminated.*

- **Inverted microscope with image capture.** An inverted microscope is an optical microscope configured with the objectives positioned below the stage in order to observe live cells adhering to the bottom of a culture vessel. In the biological laboratory, these systems are generally equipped with phase contrast (which allows visualization of live, unstained cells) in combination with fluorescence (for visualization of fluorescent proteins or dyes). Images captured using a CCD (charge-coupled device) camera attached to the microscope may be analyzed using computer software.

- **Hemacytometer.** A hemacytometer is a device used to count cells in suspension as a means of determining the density of cells within the suspension. It is a thick, glass slide etched with counting grids. A coverslip is placed over the counting grids and then a small sample of the cell suspension is injected into the narrow space between. With the aid of a microscope, the cells that reside over a defined area of the grid are counted. This cell count can be translated into density within the suspension (in cells per milliliter) because the dimensions of the counting chamber are known. A detailed protocol for counting cells with a hemacytometer can be found in Section 3.6.8.

1.4 Commonly Used Consumable Items

The strict requirement for sterility and the need to prevent cross-contamination during cell culture protocols make it convenient to use disposable supplies. These consumable items are sterilized by different means, depending upon the materials from which they are made. Generally, these items are available in a wide variety of sizes and accuracies to suit experimental requirements.

- **Serological pipettes.** These pipettes are typically used with pipette aids to handle serum, growth media, buffers, and other aqueous solutions with volumes ranging from ~0.2 to 100 mL. Sterile serological pipettes are available individually wrapped and therefore are very convenient for use in the BSC. Common sizes of serological pipettes are 1, 2, 5, 10, 25, and 50 mL and most brands are color coded for easy size selection. *Materials:* commonly, polystyrene; *sterilization:* γ-radiation.

- **Pasteur pipettes.** Pasteur pipettes are glass pipettes with long, fine tips that must be attached to a rubber bulb or vacuum source for pipetting. They are inexpensive and, due to excellent chemical resistance, are especially suited for transferring organic solvents and reagents when volume accuracy is not required. These pipettes are most commonly used for liquid aspiration into a vacuum trap. Pasteur pipettes should be disposed of in broken glass disposal. *Materials:* glass; *sterilization:* autoclave in stainless steel or polycarbonate canisters.

- **Pipette tips.** Pipette tips are used with micropipettes to handle small liquid volumes (<1 mL). They are also appropriate for handling certain organic solvents due to the enhanced chemical resistance of the material. *Materials:* commonly, polypropylene; *sterilization:* autoclave (γ-radiated packs are available for purchase).

- **Weighing supplies.** These include weigh boats, weigh paper, and disposable spatulas. *Materials:* paper or polystyrene; *sterilization:* available for purchase in sterile format.

- **Tissue culture vessels.** Tissue culture vessels come in a variety of shapes and sizes and include petri dishes, flasks, and multiwell plates. The surfaces of these vessels have generally been treated by oxygen plasma to enhance cell attachment. Use only vessels that are designated for tissue culture use unless "nontreated" vessels are specifically called for in an experiment.* *Materials:* commonly, polystyrene; *sterilization:* γ-radiation.

- **Conical centrifuge tubes.** Disposable conical centrifuge tubes are used for centrifugation of cells and are convenient liquid containers for volumes ranging from ~5 to 50 mL. *Materials:* commonly, polypropylene or polyethylene; *sterilization:* γ-radiation.

- **Microcentrifuge tubes and vials.** Small vials (such as 0.5 or 1.5 mL microcentrifuge tubes) are often used for liquid storage (i.e., aliquots of reagent stock). Cryogenic vials (cryovials) are resistant to the extremely low temperature of liquid nitrogen (–196°C) and are used for storage of cells. The screw cap of cryogenic vials often has an O-ring to seal the content. *Materials:* commonly, polypropylene; *sterilization:* γ-radiation or autoclave.

- **Autoclave supplies.** This category of supplies includes sterilization pouches and autoclave indicator tape. Small equipment such as scissors, forceps, spatulas, stir bars, etc., can be sealed in sterilization pouches, autoclaved, and stored within the pouch to maintain sterility. Most sterilization pouches include an indicator to show whether or not the item has been properly sterilized. Bottles, beakers covered with foil, boxes, and other closed items can be autoclaved without placing them in pouches. In this case, autoclave indicator tape should be affixed prior to sterilization. The white stripes on the tape will turn black when sterilization conditions are met.

- **Filters for liquid sterilization.** Liquids that contain heat labile molecules such as proteins or drugs cannot be autoclaved. Instead, they can be sterilized by filtration. The pore size of sterile filters is typically 0.22 μm (or 0.1 μm for more stringent requirements), a size that does not allow passage of microbes. Small volumes of liquid (typically, <50 mL) can be sterile filtered with syringe-tip filters that fit to the end of sterile plastic syringes. Larger liquid volumes are typically handled using bottle-top filter units connected to a vacuum source. *Materials:* various plastic materials; *sterilization:* γ-radiation.

---

* Petri dishes and multiwell plates have loose-fitting lids to allow gas exchange with the environment. For the same reason, flasks are available with vented caps. If you use flasks without a vent, it is necessary to loosen the cap before putting the flask into the incubator.

- **Syringes and needles.** Different size syringes are convenient to have on hand for filter sterilizing liquids of various volumes. A box of medium gauge needles (e.g., 19–21) may also be useful to stock.

- **Disposable scalpel blades.** Scalpel blades are available in different shapes. The choice of which shape to use is primarily a personal preference; however, it is important that the shape of the blade be compatible with the handle size(s) available in the lab.

References

Skalak, R., and C. F. Fox. 1988. *Tissue engineering.* New York: Liss.

Xian, W. 2009. *A laboratory course in biomaterials.* Boca Raton, FL: CRC Press/Taylor & Francis.

Chapter 2

Lab Safety

2.1 Biosafety

Biosafety refers to the safe handling of biological agents including bacteria, recombinant DNA, human blood, and mammalian cells. The emphasis of biosafety is on the safety of personnel as opposed to protecting the sample from being infected. Cells can harbor the same viruses, such as hepatitis and HIV, and other microbes that infect humans. Therefore, it is important to prevent transmission of potentially infectious agents from the cells to the lab personnel. Safety measures include applying special practices, using personal protective and safety equipment, and working in a properly equipped facility.

The Centers for Disease Control and Prevention (CDC) have published guidelines that categorize biosafety into four levels. The CDC publication, *Biosafety in Microbiological and Biomedical Laboratories* (BMBL), should be carefully read by anyone working with biohazardous materials (Chosewood and Wilson 2009). According to the CDC, biosafety level 1 (BSL-1) is limited to working with "well-characterized agents not known to consistently cause disease in immunocompetent adult humans, and [that] present minimal potential hazard to laboratory personnel and the environment" (Chosewood and Wilson 2009). Biosafety level 2 (BSL-2) involves "agents that pose moderate hazards to personnel and the environment" (Chosewood and Wilson 2009). Any BSL-1 or above lab must have a sign incorporating the universal biohazard symbol at the entrance (Figure 2.1). The experiments included in this book are classified as BSL-1; however, you may be working in a lab where BSL-2 work is also performed. Check with your instructor regarding the biosafety level so that you can follow the appropriate guidelines.

2.2 Safety Equipment and Engineering Controls

General safety equipment, including an eyewash, emergency shower, spill kit, first aid kit, and fire extinguisher, must be readily available in all lab environments. To use an eyewash, hold the eyelids open and flush for a minimum of 15 minutes while rotating the eyeball around in all directions. To use an emergency shower, remove

Figure 2.1
The universal biohazard symbol.

contaminated clothing and flush the affected area for a minimum of 15 minutes. It is critical to use the eyewash and shower immediately after exposure; any delay may result in irreparable tissue damage. Familiarize yourself with your surroundings. In case of emergency, know the location of the nearest eyewash station, emergency shower, hand wash station, first aid kit, spill kit, fire extinguisher, and exit. The path to these must remain unobstructed at all times. It is also important to be aware of the nearest telephone and emergency contact telephone numbers.

Through engineering controls, the lab infrastructure also helps prevent or minimize exposure to chemical and physical hazards. Examples of engineering controls typically found in a tissue-engineering lab include lab ventilation, chemical fume hoods, and biosafety cabinets (BSCs). Lab ventilation reduces exposure to airborne contaminants by directing airflow away from public areas, such as the hallway outside the lab, and by continuously circulating fresh air into the lab. Chemical fume hoods clear hazardous dusts, gases, vapors, and fumes generated within the hood so that they do not escape into the lab environment. BSCs use high-efficiency particulate air (HEPA) filters to remove airborne particulates and aerosols that may spread biohazardous materials.

2.3 Personal Protective Equipment

Personal protective equipment (PPE) includes clothing and accessories worn on the body that help prevent exposure to chemical or physical hazards. Your institution and instructors create a safe environment for you to work in; however, it is ultimately your responsibility to protect yourself. The best way to avoid an unfortunate safety incident is to be informed and to utilize the PPE available to you.

The PPE commonly available in tissue-engineering labs includes disposable latex or nitrile gloves, cryogloves, autoclave gloves, lab coats, safety glasses, and face shields. In BSL-1 labs and above, disposable gloves must be worn to protect hands from hazardous exposure (Chosewood and Wilson 2009). Latex gloves are relatively inexpensive but have poor chemical resistance and can cause allergic reactions. Nitrile gloves have much better chemical resistance and should be worn when handling organic solvents or caustic reagents. Another advantage of nitrile over latex is that a tear or hole is much easier to detect in a nitrile glove because it will rip when punctured. Gloves should be changed when their integrity is compromised or when they become contaminated.

Special gloves should be used when handling extremely hot or cold items. Cryogloves should be worn when working with liquid nitrogen because they are thick, long, and provide needed protection against the extreme cold. Cryogloves generally have an exterior waterproof or water-resistant layer and a thick, insulating liner. Autoclave gloves, made typically from thick cotton cloth, should be worn when removing items from an autoclave or oven. These gloves insulate hands from the heat only when dry; do not handle wet or damp items from the autoclave.

Lab coats or gowns are recommended to prevent contamination of clothing in BSL-1 labs and are required in BSL-2 or above labs (Chosewood and Wilson 2009). Safety glasses or face shields should be worn whenever there is a potential to splash hazardous material. Before leaving the lab, remove all PPE and wash your hands, even if you were wearing gloves while working.

2.4 Material Safety Data Sheets

Students, employees, and emergency personnel who are exposed to potentially hazardous materials need convenient access to safety information about these materials. Local and federal regulations govern how this information is provided. In the United States, the Occupational Safety and Health Administration (OSHA) requires chemical manufacturers and importers to provide a material safety data sheet (MSDS) for all potentially hazardous materials. The MSDS summarizes the procedures for safe handling, storage, and disposal of these materials.

Although the format and content may vary, similar documents exist throughout the world. Many of the chemicals and reagents used in the following experiments may pose serious health, fire, and physical hazards if used improperly. Therefore, to ensure your safety, it is necessary to review the MSDS carefully for each chemical or reagent that you plan to use. According to OSHA regulations, each MSDS must provide the following information (US Department of Labor, Occupational Safety and Health Administration):

- **Chemical identity:** for a single substance, the name of the hazardous chemical as it appears on the label and its common name; for a chemical mixture, the common name of the mixture and the chemical and common names of each ingredient known to be hazardous
- **Physical and chemical characteristics,** which may include boiling point, melting point, specific gravity, solubility, appearance, and odor
- **Physical hazards,** including potential for fire, explosion, and reactivity; may also include fire-fighting procedures, materials or conditions to avoid, and hazardous by-products
- **Health hazards,** including routes of entry into the body, exposure limits, signs and symptoms of exposure, recognition of the material as a carcinogen, and medical conditions aggravated by exposure to the chemical

- **Precautions for safe handling and use,** including protective measures while working with contaminated equipment, procedures for cleaning up spills, and precautions for handling and storage
- **Control measures,** including recommended personal protective equipment, engineering controls, and hygienic practices
- **Emergency and first aid procedures** for dealing with inhalation, ingestion, or contact with eyes or skin
- **Name and emergency contact information** for the party responsible for preparing the MSDS, such as the manufacturer or importer
- **Date** that the MSDS was prepared or updated

MSDSs are available from multiple, convenient sources. An MSDS for each chemical housed within a lab should be readily available to personnel *within the lab*. Hard copies of these MSDSs should be centrally located (for example, bound within a spiral notebook) and displayed prominently. Alternatively or in addition, electronic copies of the MSDSs can be stored on lab computers. Regardless of the format, the MSDSs must be easy to access from the lab in an emergency. MSDSs may also be found online because many chemical suppliers provide an MSDS on their website for each product they sell. When searching online, keep in mind that many chemicals have similar names and that formulations of a chemical may vary from supplier to supplier. To find the correct MSDS, visit the website of the company that supplied the chemical you are using and search for the catalog number. The catalog number is typically found on the label and/or your instructor may provide a chemical inventory that includes catalog numbers.

You are responsible for your own safety and the safety of those around you. It is *essential* to review all relevant MSDSs before beginning an experiment. Ask your instructor where the MSDSs are located within your lab and how to access the same information prior to arriving in the lab.

2.5 Safety Training

Institution, local, and/or federal regulations may mandate completion of specific safety training before you are able to enter the lab to work. Completing this training and understanding the precautions that you should take will ensure that you are comfortable while working in the lab and that you will ultimately be more successful with your experiments.

2.6 Waste Disposal

Waste commonly generated in a tissue-engineering lab includes biohazardous, chemical, and nonhazardous waste. *Biohazardous waste* is material of biological origin, such as tissue, cells, or serum, as well as any solid or liquid that has come into contact with these materials. *Chemical waste* includes solids and liquids with one or more components that may pose a health, fire, environmental, or other hazard. MSDSs should be reviewed to determine the specific hazards associated with a chemical or reagent. Some MSDSs will indicate that the hazards are not fully characterized. In this case, it is recommended to handle, collect, and dispose of the material as you would for a dangerous chemical. *Nonhazardous waste* includes paper products that have not come into contact with any biologic material as well as some commonplace chemicals (e.g., NaCl).

It is essential to observe institutional, local, and federal guidelines for collecting and disposing of waste. In many institutions, chemical and biohazardous waste that is generated in individual labs is collected, stored temporarily in the lab, and then periodically transferred to a company that specializes in hazardous waste disposal. During this process, the waste is handled by many different people; therefore, it is important to label all waste collected clearly and accurately. Always ask your instructor if you are not sure about how to collect, dispose of, or label any waste.

The following is a list of different categories of waste and corresponding disposal methods typically used in tissue-engineering labs (Figure 2.2):

- **Biohazard liquid waste.** Used media, serum, and other liquids that are biohazards, but *not* chemical hazards, can be collected in a labeled beaker throughout an experiment. At the end of the experiment, the liquid waste should be treated with 10% bleach for 30 minutes and then poured down the drain with running water. It is essential to treat the waste for the proper length of time to ensure that it is completely decontaminated. Alternatively, when working in the biosafety cabinet, liquid biohazardous waste can be aspirated with a Pasteur pipette and collected in a glass vacuum flask. Before the flask reaches two-thirds full, the contents should be disposed of properly. Depending on institutional guidelines, bleach can be added to the flask before connecting it to the vacuum source so that waste is treated immediately when aspirated into the flask. If your institution does not allow bleach in the vacuum trap, the liquid waste should be treated with 10% bleach for 30 minutes and then poured down the drain with running water.
- **Biohazard solid waste.** Large containers lined with two autoclavable bags displaying the universal biohazard symbol should be used to dispose of biohazardous items such as empty tissue culture flasks, multiwell plates, and contaminated gloves. Biohazardous waste is double bagged to lessen the chances of the waste puncturing a hole through the bag. For this same reason, some institutions require pipette tips and serological pipettes to be treated as sharps.
- **Biohazard sharps waste.** Heavy-duty, puncture-proof plastic bins displaying the universal biohazard symbol should be used to dispose of sharp or breakable biohazardous items such as Pasteur pipettes, glass coverslips, and needles. If small amounts of nonhazardous sharps are generated in the lab, including razors or dermal punches used to cut nonbiologic materials, the same container can also be used to dispose of these items. To avoid injury, it is important that you do not overfill the bin. A sharps bin is too full if it is necessary to push an item into the bin because it does not fall in freely. Once a bin is full, snap the lid closed and ask your instructor where to store it for pickup.
- **Chemical waste (liquid and solid).** Used chemicals such as DNA-binding dyes, solvents, and strong acids or bases should be collected in designated containers that

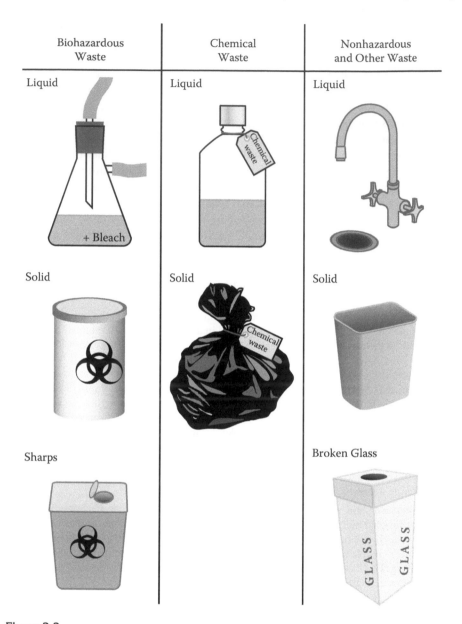

Figure 2.2
Schematic of the different waste containers and disposal methods typically found in a tissue engineering lab. Biohazardous waste includes material of biological origin and any liquid, solid, or sharp item that has come into contact with material of biological origin. Chemical waste includes liquids and solids that may pose health, fire, environmental, or other hazards. Nonhazardous waste includes paper products that have not come into contact with any biologic material and some commonplace chemicals. Broken glass containers are specifically for clean, nonhazardous broken glassware unless marked with a biohazard symbol. Ask your instructor if you are not sure about how to collect, dispose of, or label any waste.

are labeled according to institutional guidelines. As a general rule, do not mix liquid wastes and solid wastes if possible. The waste containers should be stored in a designated location within the lab and disposed of following institutional guidelines.

- **Nonhazardous liquid waste.** Institutional and local guidelines must be strictly followed for sink disposal. In general, only small amounts of nonhazardous inorganic salts, acids, and bases can be flushed down the sink with large amounts of water. *Remember to pretreat biohazardous liquid waste with bleach prior to disposal.*

- **Nonhazardous solid waste.** Items that have not come in contact with any biological materials, such as the wraps for serological pipettes or tissue paper used for disinfection with 70% alcohol, can be discarded in the regular trash.

- **Broken glass.** Clean, nonhazardous broken glassware such as Pasteur pipettes, beakers, etc., should be collected in a designated plastic-lined sharps container clearly marked as "broken glass disposal." Residual chemicals or reagents should be removed from the glassware before disposal.

References

Chosewood, L. C., and D. E. Wilson. 2009. *Biosafety in microbiological and biomedical laboratories,* ed. US Department of Health and Human Services.

US Department of Labor, Occupational Safety and Health Administration. Hazard communication. In *Toxic and hazardous substances.* Washington, DC: Author.

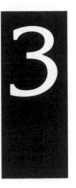

Chapter 3

Essential Lab Skills for Tissue Engineers

3.1 Introduction

This chapter provides an overview of essential lab skills and equipment operation. In addition to mastering these essential skills and equipment operation, it is important to come to each lab prepared and to take extensive notes during each experiment. Your time in the lab will be significantly more productive, enjoyable, and successful if you have *studied* the protocols, done the necessary calculations, and completed prelab questions.

These preparations should be documented in your lab notebook, which also serves as a reminder of what you did in the lab and, perhaps more importantly, is a record to everyone else of the results that you obtained and exactly how you got those results. The notebook should be written in such a manner that it is legible to other individuals and accurately reflects the objective of the experiment, the details of your actions in the lab, and the exact data that you obtained. Do not forget to include all pertinent information—including methods that proved to be unsuccessful! Finally, keep in mind that there is often more than one way of executing a lab protocol. Alternate information and lab exercises can be found in a related chapter of *A Laboratory Course in Biomaterials,* an excellent companion book to this text (Xian 2009).

3.2 Using an Electronic Balance

Using a top-loading electronic balance to weigh reagents is fairly straightforward. Place a weigh boat or weigh paper on the platen, tare (zero) the balance, add the sample to the weighing boat/paper, and read the displayed weight. Observe the following guidelines when weighing samples:

- **Range.** Each balance has a maximum capacity and "readability." Do not weigh out a sample that is outside the range of the balance. Similarly, select a balance with the required precision.

- **Leveling.** It is important to level an *analytic balance* before using it. Check the bubble level (window in which an air bubble is sealed in water). If the bubble is not centered, adjust the screws on the feet of the balance until the bubble is centered.

- **Weighing powder sample.** When weighing a powder sample, use a spatula or scoop to transfer the powder to a weigh boat (or paper) positioned in the center of the balance. When the target weight is near, lightly tap the wrist of the hand holding the spatula to allow a small amount of powder to fall into the weigh boat. Continue this gentle tapping process until the target weight is achieved. *Do not return extra powder from the weigh boat back to the stock container.*

- **Cleaning up.** Use a lab tissue or designated brush to clean up any spilled sample. Tare the empty balance.

3.3 Measuring and Transferring Liquids

You should select the appropriate method for measuring and/or transferring from one container to another depending on the volume of liquid, sterility requirements, and required accuracy and precision. The most common tools for measuring and transferring liquids in a tissue-engineering lab are graduated cylinders, volumetric flasks, pipette aids in conjunction with serological pipettes, micropipettes, and transfer pipettes. The markings on beakers and conical tubes are very approximate and these should not be used to measure liquids.

3.3.1 Graduated Cylinders and Volumetric Flasks

Graduated cylinders and volumetric flasks are liquid measuring devices mainly used for making solutions or measuring volumes > 100 mL. Volumetric flasks are used when very high accuracy is needed. For the solutions described in this manual, graduated cylinders are sufficient for making solutions. Graduated cylinders may or may not be autoclavable and it is generally good practice to avoid pouring solutions when working in a sterile environment, such as in a biosafety cabinet (BSC). For these reasons, graduated cylinders are not commonly used for measuring and transferring liquid when performing cell and tissue culture.

3.3.2 Pipette Aids

A pipette aid is a device that is used with serological pipettes to transfer liquid volumes ranging from <1 to ~100 mL. Prior to use, an unused serological pipette is attached to the nosepiece of the pipette aid. Most pipette aids are electrical and are controlled by two buttons on the handle. The top button is depressed to draw liquid up into the serological pipette while the lower button is depressed to eject liquid out of the pipette. Flow rate is proportional to the degree that the button is pushed. Pay attention to the following when using a pipette aid:

- **Select the correct size serological pipette.** It is a good rule of thumb to choose a pipette that most precisely measures the desired volume. Specifically, never use a pipette if the desired volume is <10% of the maximum capacity for a given pipette *and* do not exceed the intended maximum capacity. For example, do not use a 5 mL pipette to measure <500 µL or to measure 7 mL. Once you have mastered the use of a pipette aid, you may find it occasionally convenient to exceed the maximum intended capacity; however, you risk drawing liquid into the nosepiece of the pipette aid as described next.

- **Aspirating.** Liquid should be drawn up smoothly into the pipette. Allowing the liquid to "spring" through the opening of the pipette risks overshooting the pipette's maximum capacity and drawing liquid into the nosepiece of the pipette aid. *Never draw liquid into the nosepiece of the pipette aid as it will contaminate the filter, block air flow, and interfere with pipette aid operation.* Most serological pipettes have a white, fiber plug at the top to help protect against overfilling. In most cases, however, these plugs do not prevent overfilling but are useful as a visual indication of whether or not the liquid passed through the plug and into the nosepiece. If liquid is drawn into the nosepiece, you should immediately stop what you are doing and check that the filter is clean before proceeding. If contaminated, the filter should be replaced immediately.

- **Dispensing.** Rest the tip of the serological pipette against the inner wall of the receptacle (if possible) and deliver the liquid smoothly by pressing the lower button on the handle.

- **Pipetting organic solvent.** Glass serological pipettes must be used to pipette organic solvents as many of these reagents will dissolve pipettes made of polystyrene. You can distinguish a glass pipette by the weight compared to polystyrene pipettes (glass is heavier and will "clink" when bounced on a hard surface). Glass pipettes may be either reusable or disposable.

3.3.3 Micropipettes

Micropipettes, also called micropipetters or simply pipettes, are piston-driven air displacement devices used to transfer liquid volumes typically in the range of 0.5–1000 µL with high precision and accuracy. The percent error can be as low as <0.5% or as high as 5% depending on the micropipette used and the desired volume. A typical set of micropipettes includes one specifically for small volumes (e.g., 1–10 or 2–20 µL), one for intermediate volumes (e.g., 20–100 or 50–200 µL), and one for larger volumes (e.g., 200–1000 µL). For convenience, researchers name pipettes based on the largest volume they are rated to measure. Specifically, a pipette capable of measuring up to 20 µL is called a "P20" and a pipette capable of measuring up to 1000 µL is called a "P1000." Specialized micropipettes are available for larger or smaller volumes, and multichannel pipettes (e.g., 8 or 12 channels) are available for high-throughput applications such as microplate assays. Micropipettes may have different designs but there are common features for operation (Figure 3.1):

- **Handle.** Hold the pipette with the handle firmly in your hand.
- **Plunger.** Use your thumb to depress the plunger for initial uptake and subsequent delivery of the liquid sample. There are two stops when pushing down the plunger. For delivery of the bulk volume, press the plunger to the first stop. To deliver the residual liquid, press the plunger to the second stop.

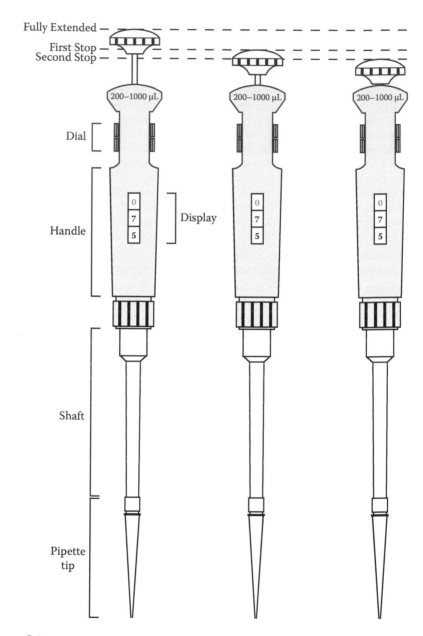

Figure 3.1

Schematic of a micropipette. The plunger is used to withdraw and eject a liquid sample from the pipette tip. There are two stops when pushing down the plunger; the first stop delivers the bulk of the liquid while the second delivers residual liquid. The dial sets the desired volume of the liquid (in microliters), which is shown on the display.

- **Volume adjustment dial.** Turn the dial to set the desired volume of the liquid to be delivered. For greatest accuracy, turn the dial past the desired volume setting and then turn it back down to the correct setting.

- **Display.** The unit for the set volumes is microliters (µL). It is important to be aware of the location of the decimal place on the dial readout. If the *most significant digit* is a different color than the others, this implies that there is a trailing 0 that is not displayed. For example, the P1000 pipette in Figure 3.1 reads 750 µL. If the *least significant digit* is a different color than the others, this implies there is a missing decimal point. For example, the pipette in Figure 3.2 reads 120.3 µL.

- **Shaft.** Disposable tips can be attached to the bottom of the shaft by firmly pushing the pipette down into the tip.

- **Tip ejector button.** To eject a used tip, point the tip toward the waste container and release it by pressing the ejector button with your thumb.

There are different techniques for using a micropipette to transfer liquid from one container to another. The following techniques are recommended depending on the volume of the liquid to be transferred and the degree of liquid viscosity (nonviscous, viscous, or foamy):

- **Forward pipetting.** The forward technique is typically used for nonviscous (aqueous) liquid. Depress the plunger to the first stop and release to draw liquid into the tip. Wipe the tip against the liquid container to remove excess liquid from the tip exterior. In the

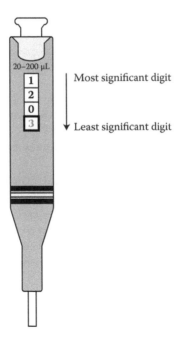

Figure 3.2
A representative 200 µL volume micropipette. The vertical numeric display indicates that the volume adjustment has been set to measure 120.3 µL (maximum volume transfer for this pipette is 200 µL).

new receptacle, press the plunger to the first stop to deliver the liquid. After a moment or two, press the plunger to the second stop to empty the tip. Release the plunger and eject the tip into the appropriate waste container.

- **Reverse pipetting.** The reverse technique is suitable for transferring viscous or foamy liquids, or small volumes. Examples of viscous or foamy liquids include solutions containing glycerol, protein, or detergents. To pipette using the reverse technique, press the plunger all the way to the second stop, then release slowly to draw liquid into the tip. Wipe the tip against the liquid container to remove excess liquid from the tip exterior. To deliver the liquid, press the plunger to the first stop and hold for 1 or 2 s. The remaining liquid should be released back into the original liquid container or discarded. Remember to pipette slowly to avoid bubble formation.

Observe the following guidelines when using a micropipette:

- Select the correct pipette. Do not use a micropipette outside its designated range; otherwise, it could be damaged mechanically. When the volume fits the ranges of several different micropipettes, select the pipette with the smallest (and therefore most accurate and precise) range. For example, to pipette a volume of 18.2 µL, use a 20 µL micropipette rather than a 100 µL micropipette.
- Use filter or barrier tips when contamination from liquid transfer is possible.
- *Never* allow liquid to flow into the micropipette barrel. This will lead to cross contamination between samples and damage the micropipette. To avoid this, pipette liquid slowly and do not tilt the micropipette too far from a vertical position when liquid is in the tip. Never hold a micropipette horizontally when it contains liquid.
- Press and release the plunger smoothly. Do not allow the plunger mechanism to snap back.
- When loading a pipette tip onto the tip cone, it is not necessary to use significant force. A light tap or two on the tip rack is generally sufficient to ensure that the tip is firmly attached.
- When aspirating liquid, do not plunge the pipette tip into the liquid; submerge it only slightly beneath the surface. Hold the pipette at a slight angle (~30°–40° off-vertical position) to ensure the greatest degree of accuracy.
- When dispensing liquid, orient the pipette tip against the inner wall of the receptacle for a steady and smooth delivery of the liquid.
- Change the tip after each use. Never return a used tip into a sterile liquid container.
- Make sure the instrument is clean. When you have completed your experiment, wipe away any moisture or soiled spots on the shaft exterior. If the micropipette has been used to handle hazardous materials, make sure that no residue is left behind.
- Store micropipettes with the volume adjustment to the highest setting. This will prevent the spring inside the micropipette from being compressed for a long period of time and help maintain accuracy.

3.3.4 Pasteur Pipettes and Disposable Transfer Pipettes

Glass Pasteur pipettes and disposable, plastic transfer pipettes serve the same function—to transfer small volumes (<10 mL) from one container to another when accuracy is not required. Pasteur pipettes are attached to a rubber bulb prior to use while transfer pipettes have a built-in bulb.

3.4 Preparing Buffers and Other Solutions

During the course of experimentation, you will need to make solutions from solid chemicals or more concentrated solutions. When preparing solutions, use clean glassware and disposable or autoclaved measuring instruments. Buffers or media containing heat-labile proteins should be sterile filtered (syringe filters for small volumes; bottle-top flask filters for larger volumes). Other solutions can be sterilized by autoclaving. Most commonly, solutions are made in deionized water (dH_2O) or phosphate-buffered saline (PBS), but it is critical to specify what the solvent or diluent should be when writing a protocol. If the protocol you are using is ambiguous, ask your instructor for clarification.

Different notations are used to express the concentrations of solutions; some notations should be familiar to you from general chemistry lab but others are probably unfamiliar. The following sections summarize these common methods for expressing solution concentrations. An excellent reference for additional information is *Lab Math: A Handbook of Measurements, Calculations, and Other Quantitative Skills for Use at the Bench* (Adams 2003).

3.4.1 Making Solutions from Solid Chemical Stock

When a solution is made by dissolving a solid (i.e., solute) in a specific volume of liquid (i.e., solvent), the resulting concentration is commonly expressed in one of three different ways:

1. **Weight of solute per volume of solution (e.g., mg/mL).** From this type of description, it is relatively straightforward to make a solution; however, you must remember to account for the volume of the solute. Specifically, if you are making 500 mL of a solution, add the solvent to the solute until the *total volume* is 500 mL. If you add 500 mL of the solvent to the solute, the final volume of the solution will be >500 mL.

2. **Moles of solute per liter of solution (e.g., mol/L, *M*, m*M*, etc.).** When making a solution from this type of description, it is essential that you check the molecular weight (MW) against the value reported on the chemical's bottle because chemicals are available in formats with different MWs. For example, calcium chloride anhydrous (MW = 111) has a different molecular weight than calcium chloride dihydrate (MW = 147). Either compound can be used to make a calcium chloride solution; however, you must account for the mass of the water (or lack thereof) when weighing the chemical on the balance. As in the preceding case, you must also account for the volume of the solute in the final solution volume.

3. **Percentage (e.g., 3%).** A 1% solution (weight/volume, w/v) is defined as 1 g of solute in 100 mL of solution. Applying this definition, it is possible to convert the concentration of a solution reported in percentage to milligrams per milliliter.

3.4.2 Making Solutions from More Concentrated Solutions

High-concentration solutions may be more stable and take up less space in the lab. As such, frequently used reagents may be stored at a high concentration and then diluted as needed to the concentration at which they are used in a protocol ("working solution"). Instructions for diluting a stock solution to achieve a working solution are typically given in one of three ways:

1. **Ratio (e.g., 1:50).** For a 1:50 dilution, mix 1 part of the concentrated stock solution with 49 parts of the diluent.

2. **Multiple of the working concentration (e.g., 50X).** The working concentration of a solution is, by definition, 1X. The concentration of the stock solution can be given as some multiple of the working concentration (e.g., double, 5 times, 10 times). A 10X stock solution must be diluted to 10 times its volume to achieve a 1X concentration. This type of description is very convenient. To make a 1X solution, divide the volume of the 1X solution that you desire by the "X" factor. The result is the amount of stock solution that should be diluted up to the total volume. For example, make 100 mL of a 1X solution from a 25X solution by diluting 100/25 mL = 4 mL of the 25X solution with 96 mL of diluent. The disadvantage to this notation is that there is no indication of the absolute concentration (e.g., M or g/mL) of the solution.

3. **Percentage (e.g., 3%).** A 1% solution (volume/volume, v/v) is defined as 1 mL of the concentrated solution diluted to 100 mL with the diluent.

3.5 Basic Microscope Operation

When working with cell cultures, it is crucial to observe and monitor living cells. An inverted phase contrast microscope is used for such a purpose. Although different models of microscopes will exhibit unique features, the underlying principles of operation are the same. Pay close attention to your instructor's demonstration and be sure to consult the manufacturer's instruction manual for more detailed information.

3.5.1 Microscope Selection

Is the microscope appropriate for the type of sample that you wish to examine visually? If you are assessing cell culture samples or other vessels containing liquid, you must use an "inverted" microscope, meaning that the objective lenses are located *beneath* the stage. With this type of system, you must be careful to avoid spilling any liquid onto the stage or particularly onto the lenses below the stage as they can be easily damaged. If you are assessing fixed cell samples (i.e., no liquid; fixed to a thin microscope slide), you can use either an inverted system or an "upright" microscope, meaning that the objectives are located *above* the stage. There is less working distance available with an upright microscope and, for this reason, this system is not compatible for examining samples in culture vessels.

It is also important to determine that the microscope system exhibits the appropriate spectral capabilities required for the sample of interest. Cells in culture are unstained and therefore require white light transmission with contrast capability in order to visualize. Phase contrast is a common transmission method to visualize cultured cells; the objective lenses contain phase rings that match a phase slider in the light path. Differential interference contrast (DIC), an alternative viewing capability for unstained cells, uses polarized light to provide sample contrast. Samples viewed in DIC appear flat and without the bright halo of light that surrounds samples viewed in phase contrast. Bright-field microscopy is suitable when viewing samples that have been stained with a contrast dye.

Finally, consider whether you will also need to view your samples using fluorescence. If so, the microscope should be outfitted with a fluorescent light source (e.g., mercury or xenon lamp) and fluorescent filters compatible with the excitation and emission spectra for the fluorophores being examined. When acquiring images of fluorescent samples, be sure also to acquire DIC images of the field of view as this is the transmitted light format most compatible with fluorescence overlay.

3.5.2 Turning on the System

Find the power switch of your microscope. When turning the system on, the halogen lamp (white light) is also turned on. Orient yourself with the lamp intensity dial in order to make the light source dimmer or brighter. If using fluorescence, ensure that the power supply for the fluorescent lamp is turned on. The lamp should be allowed to warm up for at least 15 minutes before use to prevent flickering of the light, which will interfere with accurately determining sample fluorescence intensity. If the microscope you are using is attached to an image acquisition system, locate the "view select rod" and ensure that the light path is directed toward the eyepieces and not the camera. Otherwise, you will not see anything when you look at your sample through the eyepieces.

3.5.3 Placing Your Sample on the Stage

Before the sample is placed on the stage, use the coarse focus knob to ensure that the objectives have been moved as far as possible from the stage. This ensures that the objectives will not be scratched when adjusting your sample, particularly if a stage adaptor (e.g., for six-well plates) is required. If your microscope is equipped with a mechanical stage, you can use the control rod to move the stage in the X- and Y-planes. The stage should be moved slowly so that culture medium inside the culture vessel does not splash.

3.5.4 Choosing the Correct Objective

Select the appropriate objective for initial sample viewing (this is usually the 4X or 10X in order to obtain the largest field of view). After rotating the objective into place, observe from the side of the microscope as you adjust the coarse focus knob to bring the lens close to the sample. This will ensure that you do not scratch the objective by rotating it into the sample inadvertently. Once the objective is close to the sample, you may observe through the eyepieces. Adjust the distance between the two eyepieces so that you view one circle rather than two overlapping circles. Also, practice using both eyes to look at your sample.

Check the sides of the objectives to learn specific information about them. Objectives may be *air lenses* (require space between the actual lens and sample for optimal viewing) or they may be *oil immersion lenses,* which require an overlay of immersion oil for direct contact with the sample vessel. *Never use oil on an air lens.* You should also determine whether an objective has a correction collar. Rotation of this collar adjusts critical lenses inside the objective, allowing compatible viewing with culture vessels of varying thickness. Inappropriate lens adjustment can interfere with working distance and resolution. For example, observe the difference when looking at adherent cells on a plastic culture dish compared to fixed cells attached to a thin glass coverslip.

3.5.5 Adjusting the Phase Slider

For phase contrast viewing, the phase annulus must be matched to the objective. This is accomplished by moving the phase slider. Typically, a phase contrast slider has one slot for each objective annulus as well as one open slot for bright field (no light contrast). Always match the appropriate slot in the slider to the objective you are using. If you prefer using DIC, there is no associated annulus ring to provide contrast. Rather, Köhler illumination must be performed in order to align the light path properly and provide optimal contrast. In this case, once the sample is in focus, the condenser must be closed and centering knobs used to center the light path. The condenser may then be opened to refill the field of view with light.

3.5.6 Adjusting the Focus

Use the fine-focus adjustment knobs on each side of the microscope to bring an image into focus. If you cannot find a focal plane, move the stage until the edge of the vessel or some other recognizable feature of the specimen comes into the field of view. Subsequently use the coarse adjustment knob to bring the image into focus and use the fine adjustment knob for optimization.

3.5.7 Changing the Objective Lens

Once you have viewed your sample at low magnification, it is often desirable to select a higher objective for a closer look. It is important that you *do not* simply rotate the objective turret to click the new objective in place. This is often the cause of scratched lenses or tipped culture vessels. Instead, use the coarse focus knob to move the objective away from the stage *before* rotating the turret. Once the new objective has been selected, refocus your sample as described in the previous section. You may need to readjust the light intensity as well as the phase slider after changing the objective.

3.5.8 Using Fluorescence Microscopy

Once you have visually examined your sample using white light, it is often desirable to examine the sample using fluorescence (e.g., examine cellular expression of transfected fluorescent protein markers). To do so, ensure that the power supply for the fluorescent lamp has been turned on and allowed to warm up for a minimum of 15 minutes. Often, a mercury or xenon lamp will flicker while warming up; therefore, you should not acquire any images during this period of time as this may interfere with determination of the sample's true fluorescence intensity values. Remember to block transmission of white light to the sample (turn off the transmitted light source or insert a blocking filter) to allow transmission of the fluorescent light only (Figure 3.3).

It is important to make sure that the appropriate fluorescent filters are in place for optimal signal excitation and collection of consequent emitted light. Remember that viewing your sample in a fluorescent light source for an extended period of time can cause photobleaching of the fluorophore that will interfere with appropriate assessment of sample fluorescence intensity.

3.5.9 Image Acquisition

A trinocular microscope is equipped with a phototube for camera attachment. In this case, a beam splitter can split the light emitted from the specimen between the eyepieces and the camera. The light may be directed entirely to the eyepieces or selectively directed to the camera (between 50% and 100%, depending on the type of microscope). It is important to adjust the view select rod to ensure redirection of light to the camera in order to acquire an image of your selected field of view. *Note: The focus for the camera may be different from that for the eyepieces, so be sure to adjust the focus in live mode on the computer screen before capturing images.* It is also important to familiarize yourself with the image capture software associated with the system you are using.

3.5.10 General Microscope Maintenance

While laboratory staff should ensure regular maintenance of teaching laboratory microscopes, there are a few things you can watch out for before using a system. Always check that the eyepieces are free of smudges. If not, they should be cleaned using 70% ethanol and *lens paper only.* Check the stage for spills or broken glass coverslips. The stage can be wiped using 70% ethanol and lab tissues. Notify your instructor if you identify broken

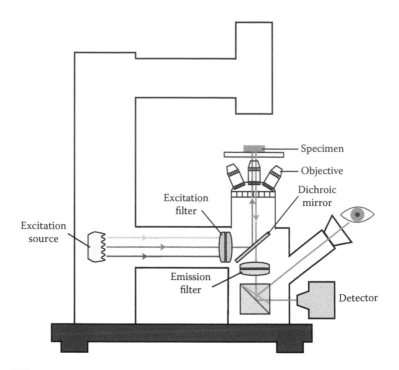

Figure 3.3

A standard inverted fluorescence microscope showing the path of light when using fluorescent illumination. Light from a high-intensity light source, such as mercury burner or laser, is sent through an *excitation* filter, which allows passage of wavelengths that will specifically illuminate the fluorophore of interest within the sample. After passing through the excitation filter, the excitation light is reflected off a dichroic mirror (also called a beam splitter) and redirected through the microscope objective toward the sample. Fluorophores within the sample absorb the excitation light and emit light at a longer wavelength. The emitted light passes through the dichroic mirror, is filtered by an emission filter, and then redirected to the eyepiece, camera, or both for visualization.

glass, which will need to be collected and carefully disposed of in the broken glass waste. Similarly, if you happen to tip your culture vessel or break a coverslip while working on the microscope, notify your instructor immediately. If either the halogen or fluorescent lamps appear to be flickering (after the initial warm-up period), it is probably an indication that the bulb should be replaced. Inform your instructor as a flickering light source can interfere with intensity measurements of the sample. Finally, when acquiring images, be sure to save the files where they will not be inadvertently deleted.

3.6 Sterile Technique and Mammalian Cell Culture

3.6.1 Disinfection

It is common practice to use a disinfectant such as 70% ethanol or 10% bleach to decontaminate work surfaces and equipment (e.g., BSCs, micropipettes, etc.). This should be done before and after protocol execution, particularly when working with cell cultures. Both of these solutions should be prepared in low-density polyethylene spray (or squirt) bottles. Bleach offers advantages in being a broad-spectrum disinfectant; however, the solution can be toxic or corrosive, so working dilutions should be made fresh every week. Ethanol is relatively fast acting and nontoxic; however, solutions can catch fire if near high-heat sources. Both disinfectants can be dangerous if splashed in the eyes.

3.6.2 Preparing the Biosafety Cabinet

When not in use, the BSC can be maintained either with the sash open and blower (which drives airflow in the cabinet) running or with the sash closed and the blower turned off (Figure 3.4). The germicidal UV lamp should be used only when no one is working in the room. It is not necessary ever to use the lamp if the following procedures are followed:

Turning on the BSC (if needed). If the fan is off and the sash is closed, the BSC must be properly vented and disinfected before use. Turn on the light inside the cabinet. Raise the sash. For some BSC models, an alarm will sound if the sash is lifted too high or pulled too low. Activate the blower and wait 15–30 minutes to allow airflow to equilibrate. Particulates accumulated within the cabinet will be removed by the HEPA filter. *Note: This step may be performed by an instructor in advance of the lab session.*

Disinfecting the BSC. Ensure that shirt sleeves are confined and remove jewelry from wrists or fingers. Wear latex or nitrile gloves and spray both hands with 70% ethanol, rubbing hands together to spread the alcohol evenly (gloves should be visibly wet). Spray the interior of the cabinet with disinfectant and use lab tissues to wipe down the work surface.

Arrange necessary items in the BCS. All items must be disinfected with 70% ethanol before being moved into the BSC. For each item that will be used in the BSC, spray the surface with 70% ethanol and wipe with a lab tissue to spread the ethanol evenly. Move the item into the BSC (the ethanol will evaporate quickly). Position the items around the perimeter of the cabinet surface. Do not block your primary work surface, which is in the middle, and do not block the air intake grill. Use the same aseptic techniques to move all other required items into the BSC.

Working in the BSC. Sit comfortably so that your arms can move freely. Do not put your elbows (or any other items) on the air intake grill as this will block airflow and increase the risk of contamination. Minimize the number of times that you remove your arms from inside the cabinet while working. In particular, assemble all required reagents and consumables inside the hood before beginning to work.

3.6.3 Media Preparation

"Base" or "basal" cell culture medium contains mostly nonperishable (or low-perish-able) small molecules such as salts, amino acids, vitamins, and carbohydrates. It is commercially available in many varieties in either powder or liquid form for use with different cell types. Base medium can be stored at 4°C for 1 year or longer.

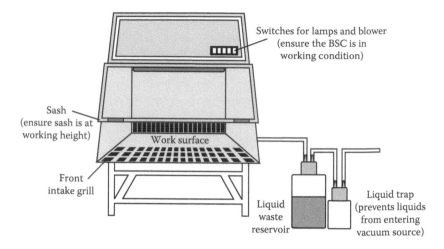

Figure 3.4
A typical BSC work environment. Use of a reservoir and liquid trap attached to a vacuum source allows liquid aspiration from samples within the sterile environment of the cabinet.

Before use in cell culture, base medium is usually supplemented with serum (which contains growth factors that promote cell proliferation) and antibiotics (which prevent microbial contamination) to make "complete" media. A combination of the antibiotics penicillin and streptomycin (P/S) is commonly used as an additive. A 100X stock solution of this mixture is widely available. Serum and antibiotics are perishable and must be frozen (−20°C) for long-term storage. Complete medium should be stored at 4°C and is generally safe to use for up to 2 weeks. As an example, the following describes how to supplement a medium base, Dulbecco's modified eagle medium (DMEM), to make complete DMEM:

1. Prepare the BSC for use by wiping it down with 70% ethanol and arranging the following inside: one 500 mL bottle of DMEM, one sterile 100 mL bottle, 50 mL of thawed serum, 5 mL of thawed 100X P/S stock, serological pipettes, and a permanent lab marker. The following items are optional depending on whether or not your instructor wants you to sterile filter the complete media: one sterile 500 mL media bottle with attached bottle-top filter and labeling tape.

2. Loosen the caps of the reagent containers but do not remove them.

3. Using a sterile serological pipette, remove 55 mL of base DMEM from the stock bottle and transfer into the sterile 100 mL bottle for storage at 4°C (this can be subsequently used as "serum-free" media in other experiments). Add 50 mL of serum and 5 mL of 100X P/S to the DMEM bottle. Make sure that the pipettes do not touch the *outside* of any bottles or tubes, or anything else inside the BSC. Cap the media bottle and *gently swirl* to mix the contents. Do not shake as you want to minimize bubble formation.

4. (Optional) Attach the sterile 500 mL media bottle with bottle-top filter to the vacuum source within the BSC. Remove the lid of the filter and pour the complete DMEM into the filter. Replace the lid on the filter and turn the vacuum source on. The complete DMEM will be drawn through the bottle-top filter into the attached sterile media

bottle. When all media have been filtered, remove the filter and discard appropriately. Securely cap the sterile media bottle.

5. Label the complete media bottle with "DMEM + 10% FBS + P/S." Use a piece of labeling tape with permanent marker if you have filtered the media into a glass bottle. Include the date of preparation and your name or initials.

6. Remove all reagents from the BSC and store them at the appropriately designated temperatures. The complete DMEM can be left in the BSC if you will be continuing with cell culture work.

3.6.4 Cryopreservation of Cells

Cells can be stored long term over liquid nitrogen, but they must be frozen in the proper media with a slow and steady drop in temperature. Adherent cells are first detached from the growth surface using trypsin and counted on a hemacytometer to determine cell concentration (refer to Sections 3.6.7 and 3.6.8). Next, the cells are pelleted in a centrifuge tube by low-speed centrifugation and resuspended in freezing medium at a density of ~1 × 10^6 cells/mL. Freezing medium contains complete culture media (80%), serum (10%), and dimethylsulfoxide (DMSO; 10%)—a cryoprotectant that reduces formation of ice crystals that can cause cell lysis. Cells are resuspended in the freezing medium by pipetting up and down carefully and then transferred in 1 mL volumes to prelabeled 2 mL cryogenic vials (Figure 3.5). The vials should be labeled using a permanent lab marker.

For freezing, the vials can be placed into the slots of a commercial cryofreezing container or into a Styrofoam tube holder and secured by inverting a second Styrofoam tube holder on top. The Styrofoam holders (or cryofreezing container) are placed into a −80°C freezer for 2–48 h to bring the cell suspension slowly down to temperature. Finally, the cryovials are transferred to a liquid nitrogen tank (−196°C) for long-term storage in the liquid vapor phase.

3.6.5 Thawing Cryopreserved Cells

Cryopreserved cells must be thawed before being plated in tissue culture vessels for experimental use. The cells will come to life when thawed. If working with adherent cells, work efficiently to prevent cells from adhering to surfaces other than the intended culture vessel.

1. Prepare the BSC for use by wiping it down with 70% ethanol and arranging the following inside: complete media, sterile T25 tissue culture flask, 15 mL conical tube, serological pipettes, and a canister of sterile Pasteur pipettes.

2. With help from your instructor, remove the vial of cells from the liquid nitrogen storage. Be sure to wear cryogloves and a face shield.

3. *Quickly* thaw the frozen vial in a 37°C water bath. Use a circular motion to swirl the contents of the vial, ensuring that the neck of the vial is kept above water level to avoid contamination.

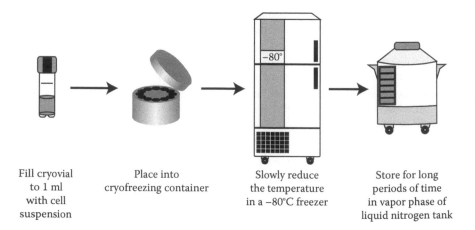

Fill cryovial   Place into   Slowly reduce   Store for long
to 1 ml   cryofreezing container   the temperature   periods of time
with cell   in a −80°C freezer   in vapor phase of
suspension   liquid nitrogen tank

Figure 3.5
Steps for slow cryopreservation of cultured cells.

4. Spray your gloves with 70% ethanol. Spray and wipe the thawed cryovial with 70% ethanol and place it inside the BSC.

5. Loosen the cap of the vial and the 15 mL conical centrifuge tube. Using a 1 mL pipette, gently pipette the contents up and down a few times inside the vial to resuspend the cells. Transfer the cell suspension into the 15 mL conical tube.

6. Using a 10 mL serological pipette, add 9 mL of complete DMEM *dropwise* to the cell suspension. It is necessary to add the media slowly in order to give the cells time to equilibrate to the osmolarity of the media, which is different from the osmolarity of the cryoprotectant they are in.

7. Gently pipette up and down a few times for complete mixing and then cap the tube.

8. Place the 15 mL tube opposite an appropriate counterbalance in a tabletop centrifuge. Centrifuge for 5 min at 250–500 *g*. When centrifugation is complete, a small white pellet should be visible at the bottom of the tube; these are the cells. Aseptically move the tube back into the BSC.

9. Loosen the cap of the 15 mL tube. Open the lid of the canister that holds the Pasteur pipettes; hold the canister horizontally and gently shake the pipettes out a bit so that you can select one pipette without touching the others. Turn on the vacuum. Connect the wide end of the Pasteur pipette to the aspirator vacuum hose inside the BSC. Carefully use the tip of the Pasteur pipette to aspirate the majority of the supernatant from the tube. *Be very careful to keep the pipette tip away from the cell pellet or it will be suctioned away.* In performing this step, you have removed the cryoprotectant, DMSO, which is harmful to live cells.

10. Remove the cap of the T25 flask.

11. Add 5 mL of complete DMEM to the tube and gently pipette up and down to resuspend the cells (make sure that no clumps of cells are visible). *Note: For some experiments, it is recommended to count an aliquot of thawed cells to determine total number of viable cells and to control cell density in the culture flask (refer to Section 3.6.8). If this is the case, use a 1 mL serological pipette to remove ~100 μL of cell suspension from the 15 mL tube and transfer to a microcentrifuge tube. Sterile microfuge tubes*

are recommended to avoid contamination of the pipette and, subsequently, the cell suspension. The cell samples used for counting will not be cultured and therefore they do not need to be kept aseptic.

12. Using the same pipette, transfer the cell suspension from the 15 mL tube into the T25 flask. Cap the flask and gently rock the medium back and forth across the width of the flask to spread the cells evenly. If the flask is not vented, loosen the cap to allow for gas exchange in the incubator.

13. Label the flask to indicate the cell line, passage number, date, and your name. You can write directly on the flask since it is disposable.

14. Transfer the flask into a 37°C CO_2 incubator.

15. Discard the cryogenic vial and the 15 mL tube into the biohazard waste. Discard the Pasteur pipette into the biohazard sharps waste. Store the complete DMEM at 4°C. Wipe down the BSC with 70% ethanol.

3.6.6 Refeeding Cell Cultures/Changing Media

As cultured cells proliferate, nutrients in the media are gradually depleted and waste accumulates. To maintain the health of the culture, the media needs to be changed every 2 or 3 days. Some culture media contain phenol red, an indicator of pH. Media that have changed color from red to yellow have overgrown and been depleted of essential nutrients or become infected and should be discarded.

1. In a 37°C water bath, warm a bottle of complete media.

2. View the cells using an inverted microscope. Note the cell morphology and extent of confluence.

3. Prepare the BSC for use by wiping it down with 70% ethanol and arranging the following inside: complete media, serological pipettes, a canister of sterile Pasteur pipettes, and the flask of cells.

4. Use a Pasteur pipette to aspirate the old medium. Keep the tip of the pipette to a corner of the flask and take care not to scratch the cells (Figure 3.6).

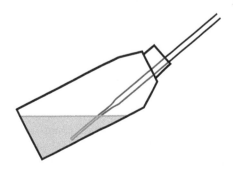

Figure 3.6
Suggested method for aspirating media from a monolayer culture so that the cell layer is not disturbed.

TABLE 3.1

Approximate Area and Recommended Media Volume for Common Tissue Culture Flasks, Dishes, and Multiwell Plates

Culture Vessel	Approximate Culture Area (cm^2)	Recommended Media Volume per Plate, Flask, or Well (mL)
T25 Flask	25	5
T75 Flask	75	15
35 mm Dish	10	2
60 mm Dish	21	4.5
100 mm Dish	57	12
150 mm Dish	154	30
6-Well plate	9.6	2
12-Well plate	3.8	0.8
24-Well plate	2.0	0.4
48-Well plate	0.9	0.2
96-Well plate	0.3	0.1

Note: The names of the dishes (35 mm, 60 mm, etc.) do not correspond to the actual dish diameter.

5. Add fresh medium to the flask. Do *not* splash the medium on the cell growth surface or the cells will be dislodged. Table 3.1 summarizes the recommended media volumes for common sizes of flasks, dishes, and multiwell plates.

6. Label the flask with the date of medium change and your initials. Move the flask back to the 37°C CO_2 incubator. Store the complete DMEM at 4°C.

3.6.7 Passaging Cell Cultures/Trypsinizing a Cell Monolayer*

Adherent cells generally grow as a monolayer in culture. When the cells proliferate to the point where there is no culture surface remaining, the culture is said to have reached *confluency*. At this density, "contact inhibition" occurs and the cells stop dividing and begin to die (within days). In addition, changes in gene regulation and expression often occur in confluent cells. For these reasons, a cell culture needs to be "passaged" or "split" *before* it reaches confluency.

Adherent cells must be detached from the growth surface before passaging can occur. This is achieved by incubating the cells in the presence of trypsin. Trypsin is a naturally occurring enzyme that cleaves side chains of the amino acids lysine and arginine. Trypsin degrades cell surface proteins, including the adhesion proteins, detaching cells from the growth surface and suspending them in the culture media.

---

* This protocol is also included as Appendix 1.

TABLE 3.2
Recommended Volume of Trypsin to Use to Release a Cell Monolayer from Common Size Flasks and Dishes

Culture Vessel	Approximate Culture Area (cm²)	Recommended Trypsin Volume to Release Cells (mL)	Recommended Trypsin Volume to Thaw (mL)
T25 Flask	25	1.0	2.0
T75 Flask	75	3.0	6.0
35 mm Dish	10	0.5	1.0
60 mm Dish	21	1.0	2.0
100 mm Dish	57	2.0	4.0

Note: Thaw at least twice the volume needed for the trypsinization so that the excess can be used for rinsing.

The cell suspension can easily be counted and/or diluted before seeding a new culture. The following protocol can be used whenever it is necessary to release cells from monolayer culture, either to passage the cells or to use the cells in an experiment. *Note: Cells in a suspension culture are not adherent and are passaged by removing a fraction of cell-containing media for further dilution into new sterile flasks.*

1. In a 37°C water bath, warm 0.25% trypsin and complete media. The volume of trypsin recommended to release cells from common culture vessels is shown in Table 3.2. Thaw at least twice the volume needed to release the cells so that the excess can be used for rinsing.

2. Prepare the BSC for use by wiping it down with 70% ethanol and arranging necessary reagents and disposables.

3. Remove the culture vessel(s) from the incubator, spray lightly with 70% ethanol, and place in the BSC.

4. Aspirate the spent medium from the culture vessel with a Pasteur pipette. Position the Pasteur pipette so the media are removed without disturbing the cell monolayer.

5. *Quickly* rinse the cell monolayer with half of the trypsin to dilute media and waste components.

6. *Quickly* and carefully aspirate this rinse solution with a Pasteur pipette.

7. Add the remaining warmed trypsin to the flask. Place the flask in the incubator.

8. Check on the cells after 2–3 min to see if they have detached. *Gently* tap on the side of the flask to release the cells. View cells under the microscope to confirm detachment. Incubate the cells for a few minutes longer if they have not detached. *Avoid exposing cells to trypsin longer than required to release them from the substrate because trypsin will damage cell surface receptors and may slow cell adhesion and spreading.*

9. Add 10 mL of complete media (with serum) to neutralize the trypsin action.

10. Thoroughly rinse the bottom and corners of the flask to release adherent cells.

11. Split, concentrate, or use cells as desired:
    a. Split the cells by dividing up the cell suspension among multiple culture vessels and then adding media to bring the volume in each vessel up to the working

volume. A sample of the cell suspension can be counted using a hemacytometer (see Section 3.6.8) to determine how to split the cells or a standard "split ratio" can be used. A typical split ratio is 1:10, which means plating the same number of cells on a surface area 10-fold larger then previously. For example, cells from a single T75 flask can be replated into ten T75 flasks.

b. To concentrate the cells, spin the suspension down for 5 min in a centrifuge at 250–500 *g*, discard the supernatant, resuspend the pellet in a small volume of media, count a sample on the hemacytometer, and adjust to desired density.

3.6.8 Counting Cells with a Hemacytometer*

A hemacytometer is a microscopic counting grid that can be used to determine the density of a cell suspension (Figure 3.7). While counting cells on a hemacytometer, it is possible to estimate the percentage of viable cells in the whole population by using a stain called trypan blue. Healthy cells with intact membranes are able to exclude trypan blue and appear colorless, while unhealthy or dead cells with disrupted plasma membranes cannot exclude the dye and appear blue. *Caution: trypan blue is carcinogenic and can be absorbed through skin. Always wear gloves when working with trypan blue and collect contaminated waste in a special waste container.*

1. Clean the hemacytometer and cover glass with 70% ethanol. Wipe with a lint-free wiper or blow dry with compressed air. Moisturize the coverslip supports with water and gently place the coverslip on top (this small amount of water will act as adhesive to hold the coverslip down) before adding cell suspension.

2. Mix the cell suspension with trypan blue:

    a. In the BSC, mix the cell suspension thoroughly to break up cell clumps and to obtain a homogenous suspension. Withdraw the entire cell suspension into a serological pipette. Eject the suspension slowly, collecting two samples (one drop each) mid-stream in separate microfuge tubes. *Note: Sterile microfuge tubes are recommended to avoid contamination of the pipette and, subsequently, the cell suspension.*

    b. Take the microfuge tubes to the lab bench; it is not necessary to keep the samples sterile since they will be discarded after the cells are counted.

    c. In another microfuge tube, mix 40 µL from one of the samples with 10 µL of trypan blue. Repeat with the second sample.

3. Load the cell/trypan blue mixtures into opposite sides on the hemacytometer:

    a. Mix the cells with trypan blue thoroughly by pipetting up and down repeatedly.

    b. Withdraw 10 µL of the first sample into a pipette.

    c. Rest the pipette tip on one of the notches of the hemacytometer (Figure 3.7).

    d. Gently depress the pipette's plunger, allowing the mixture to flow into the chamber by capillary action. Inject enough to cover the counting surface, but do not allow the chamber to overflow.

    e. Load the counting chamber on the other side with the second cell/trypan blue sample.

---

* This protocol is also included as Appendix 2.

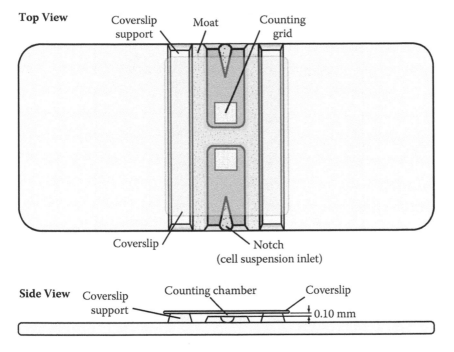

Figure 3.7
Schematic of a hemacytometer. The critical features are two precision-etched counting grids and a pre-cise distance between the coverslip and the counting grids. The space between the coverslip and the etched surface below forms a counting chamber.

4. Count the cells:

    a. Place the hemacytometer on the microscope stage.

    b. Using transmitted light and a low-powered objective (e.g., 10X), adjust the focus and hemacytometer position so that a grid pattern is clearly visible (Figure 3.8).

    c. With a hand tally counter, count and record the number of *live* cells in region 1 of Figure 3.8 (5 × 5 large squares). This region has an area of 1 mm^2. To avoid count-ing the same cell twice, follow a systematic pattern with your eyes and count cells present on the top and left border but not those on the bottom or right border (as shown in Figure 3.9).

    d. Count and record the number of *dead* cells in the same region.

    e. A good *live* cell count is between 100 and 500 cells; if the cell count is too low, then the sample may not be representative of the cell suspension. If the cell count is too high, it may be difficult to distinguish between neighboring cells. If your count falls well outside this target range, dilute or concentrate the cell suspension as needed and repeat the preceding steps. If your cell count falls within this range, count the second sample, which is already loaded onto the opposite side of the hemacytometer.

5. If the values obtained from the two grids vary significantly (>10%), the original cell suspension may not be evenly mixed and should be recounted. The process should also

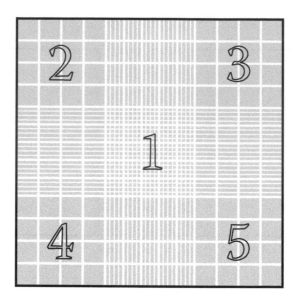

Figure 3.8
One of the two identical counting grids on a hemacytometer. Region 1 (5 × 5 large squares) is the 1 mm² area over which the cells should be counted.

be repeated if there is an abundance of clumped cells visible in the grid. Repeat steps 1–4 until reliable and repeatable counts are obtained. Average the counts.

6. Calculate the percent viability in the cell suspension:

$$\% \text{ Viability} = \frac{\text{Live Cell Count}}{(\text{Live Cell Count} + \text{Dead Cell Count})} \times 100\% \qquad (3.1)$$

7. Calculate the density of cells in the suspension from which the samples were collected (cells per milliliter). Taking into consideration the dilution by the trypan blue, the cell density is

$$\text{Live Cell Density} = 10{,}000 \times 1.25 \times N \qquad (3.2)$$

where N is the average live cell count from the two samples. *Note: If the live cell density is less than desired, centrifuge the suspension, resuspend the cell pellet in a smaller volume, and repeat the cell counts.*

8. Calculate the total number of live cells in your cell suspension:

$$\text{Total Live Cells} = \text{Live Cell Density} \times \text{Volume of Cell Suspension} \qquad (3.3)$$

9. Calculate the final suspension volume that will achieve the desired density in the cell suspension (as needed):

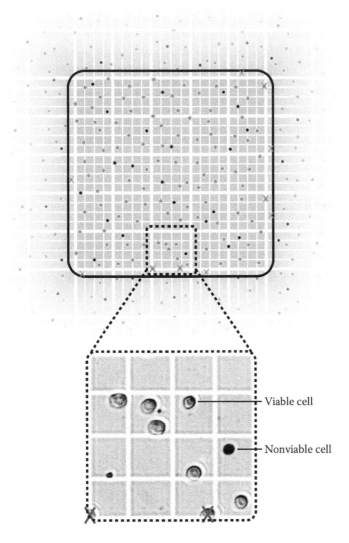

Figure 3.9
Count cells within individual squares and those touching the left and top borders. Do not count cells that touch the right and bottom borders. Counting should start from the upper right corner and "snake" back and forth until the lower right corner is reached. To determine the percentage of viable cells, count the number of viable and nonviable cells. The percentage of viable cells (82%) is the number of viable cells (98) divided by the total number of cells (120) in the field. The micrograph at the bottom illustrates how viable and nonviable cells appear under the microscope.

$$\text{Final Suspension Volume} = \frac{\text{Total Live Cells}}{\text{Desired Cell Density}} \qquad (3.4)$$

10. Bring the cell suspension up to the final volume by adding media. Mix well and use the cells as desired.

11. Carefully remove the coverslip and hold it over a trypan blue liquid waste container to spray-wash with 70% ethanol. Spray-wash the chamber slide as well. Use a lab tissue to rub mild detergent gently on the slide and coverslip to remove cellular residue, and rinse with water followed by deionized water. Place the hemacytometer and coverslip on a lab tissue to dry. Rinse the 0.5 mL microcentrifuge tube with 70% ethanol to remove residual trypan blue (the rinse goes into the trypan blue waste) and discard both this tube and the 1.5 mL microcentrifuge tube containing cell suspension into the biohazardous waste.

References

Adams, D. S. 2003. *Lab math: A handbook of measurements, calculations, and other quantitative skills for use at the bench.* Cold Spring Harbor, NY: Cold Spring Harbor Laboratory Press.

Xian, W. 2009. *A laboratory course in biomaterials.* Boca Raton, FL: CRC Press/Taylor & Francis.

Chapter 4

Isolation of Primary Chondrocytes from Bovine Articular Cartilage

4.1 Background

Cartilage is a hydrated, avascular connective tissue containing a sparse population of cells, called chondrocytes, embedded within an extensive extracellular matrix (ECM). Cartilage is classified as hyaline, elastic, or fibrocartilage based on its structure and composition.

Hyaline cartilage is found in the nasal septum, sternum, trachea, larynx, and on the articulating surfaces of long bones, where it is referred to as articular cartilage. Articular cartilage distributes loads and functions as a bearing surface in joints such as the hip and knee. The ECM of hyaline cartilage is composed primarily of collagen type II and is rich in proteoglycans. Elastic cartilage is present in the epiglottis, external ear, and larynx. The ECM of elastic cartilage contains elastin and collagen type II with less proteoglycan than hyaline cartilage. Fibrocartilage is found in the intervertebral disc, the meniscus of the knee, and at the insertion of ligaments and tendons. The ECM of fibrocartilage is composed primarily of collagen type I.

Articular cartilage is a particularly suitable clinical target for tissue engineering because cartilage disease is prevalent, cartilage exhibits limited intrinsic repair capacity, and existing pharmaceutical and surgical treatments have broad limitations. The lack of intrinsic repair capability of articular cartilage may be due to the low density of chondrocytes within the tissue (Freeman 1979). Therefore, to augment repair, cartilage tissue-engineering approaches have focused on the transplantation of chondrocytes into a defect site either alone or within a biomaterial scaffold. An early and essential step in these cell-based therapies is the isolation of chondrocytes from their surrounding ECM. As with other cell types, chondrocyte isolation is commonly accomplished through enzymatic tissue digestion (Freshney 2010). Collagenase is the enzyme used to isolate chondrocytes because collagen is the predominant protein found in the cartilage ECM.

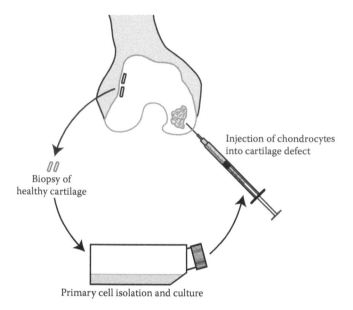

Figure 4.1
Overview of the Carticel® procedure. Small biopsies of healthy cartilage are removed from a non-load-bearing region of the patient's femur. Chondrocytes are isolated from the biopsies, expanded in number, and then injected back into the patient's knee at the site of cartilage damage.

Carticel® is a commercially available tissue-engineering treatment that involves the injection of a patient's own chondrocytes into a localized cartilage defect on the femur. Carticel was commercialized by Genzyme Corporation and, in 1997, became the first cell-based therapy to earn FDA approval (Hunziker et al. 2006). The Carticel procedure requires two surgeries separated by at least 2 weeks (Figure 4.1) (Brittberg et al. 1994; Minas and Peterson 2006; Genzyme Corporation 2011). An initial surgery is performed to obtain a small cartilage biopsy from a non-weight-bearing region of the knee joint. The biopsy is sent to Genzyme's manufacturing facility, where chondrocytes are isolated and a *primary culture* is established. Primary culture is defined as the stage of culture after isolation from tissue and before the transfer of cells from one culture vessel into another (Freshney 2010). After primary culture, the patient's cells are cryopreserved, thawed when needed, and then expanded in number.

Following cell expansion, a second surgery is performed to inject the culture-expanded chondrocytes into the cartilage defect. To help contain the cells within the defect, the chondrocytes are injected under a flap of connective tissue that is sutured to the surrounding cartilage to form a physical barrier. Patients treated with Carticel have experienced clinically meaningful improvements in pain and joint function; however, high rates of surgical revision and adverse events have been reported (Zaslav et al. 2009; Wood et al. 2006).

To verify Carticel's quality and safety, a series of tests are run prior to releasing each lot of expanded chondrocytes for implantation (Zaslav et al. 2009). One of these tests determines whether or not there are enough live chondrocytes for implantation.

Labels within figure:
Injection of chondrocytes into cartilage defect
Biopsy of healthy cartilage
Primary cell isolation and culture

The specific method used by Genzyme is proprietary; however, a widely used assay to test cell viability is commercially available. Molecular Probe's LIVE/DEAD® viability/cytotoxicity assay is a two-color fluorescence assay for simultaneously staining live and dead cells in culture or within tissue.

The two probes used in the LIVE/DEAD assay are calcein AM and ethidium homodimer (EthD-1). Calcein AM is a membrane permeable molecule that is enzymatically cleaved within the cytoplasm of viable cells to produce an intensely fluorescent dye, calcein (Molecular Probes 2005). EthD-1 enters the damaged membrane of dead cells and binds to the cell's DNA, causing a large increase in fluorescence (Molecular Probes 2005). When the dyes are used together, live cells appear green and dead cells appear red using fluorescent microscopy. In this experiment, the LIVE/DEAD assay will be used to determine the percentage of cells that are viable within a representative sample of the articular cartilage from which chondrocytes will be isolated.

4.2 Learning Objectives

The objectives of this experiment are to

- Gain experience isolating primary, mammalian cells
- Practice essential lab skills including sterile technique, counting cells using a hemacytometer, and calculations related to making and diluting solutions
- Learn to perform a widely applicable cell viability assay using fluorescence microscopy

4.3 Overview of Experiment

This experiment involves enzymatically digesting bovine cartilage to release chondrocytes from their surrounding ECM. Specifically, cartilage is minced into small pieces and digested with collagenase for 2 hours. Large pieces of undigested tissue are then separated from the isolated cells using a strainer and a monolayer culture is established with the freshly isolated chondrocytes (Figure 4.2). While the cartilage is being digested, the viability of cells within a sample of intact cartilage will be measured using the LIVE/DEAD viability assay.

4.4 Safety Notes

Use good lab practices and review all relevant MSDSs.

4.5 Materials

In addition to the general equipment and supplies, the following are needed to complete this experiment:

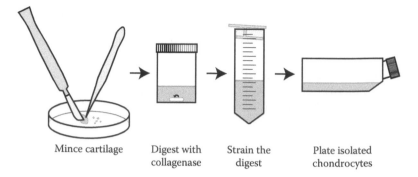

Mince cartilage   Digest with   Strain the   Plate isolated
                 collagenase   digest   chondrocytes

Figure 4.2
Overview of the chondrocyte isolation procedure including mincing the cartilage into small pieces, digesting the pieces of cartilage with collagenase, separating the isolated chondrocytes from any large pieces of undigested tissue using a strainer, and then plating the freshly isolated chondrocytes in monolayer culture.

4.5.1 Reagents and Consumables

- Fresh bovine calf articular cartilage (≥1 g wet weight)
- Chondrocyte media (recipe follows)
- Sterile specimen cup
- Collagenase P (Roche)
- 1X phosphate-buffered saline (PBS, at 25°C *and* 4°C)
- Cell strainer (40 µm mesh)
- LIVE/DEAD viability/cytotoxicity kit (Molecular Probes)
- Trypan blue

4.5.2 Equipment and Supplies

- Sterile stir bar
- Sterile forceps
- Sterile scalpel handle and blades
- Sterile spatula
- *Optional:* histology slides of hyaline, elastic, and fibrocartilage
- Microscope equipped for fluorescence and digital imaging (The product data sheet for the LIVE/DEAD viability/cytotoxicity kit has suggestions for dual emission filters for simultaneously viewing calcein [EX: 494 nm, EM: 517 nm] and EthD-1 [EX: 528 nm, EM: 617 nm].)

4.6 Recipes

250X l-proline stock (100 mM). Dissolve 0.46 g l-proline in 40 mL DMEM/F12, filter through a 0.22 µm filter, pipette 2 mL aliquots into sterile cryovials, and store at –20°C.

Chondrocyte media. Add 50 mL fetal bovine serum (FBS), 5 mL of 100X penicillin/ streptomycin (P/S), 2 mL of 250X l-proline stock, 5 mL of 200 mM l-glutamine, and 5 mL of 10 mM nonessential amino acids to 433 mL DMEM/F12.

1X PBS. Add 50 mL 10X PBS (with Ca^{2+} and Mg^{2+}) to 400 mL deionized H_2O (dH_2O). Mix well, adjust pH to 7.4 with HCl and NaOH, bring total volume to 500 mL with dH_2O, and either sterile-filter through a 0.2 μm filter or autoclave.

4.7 Methods

4.7.1 Session 1: Isolate Chondrocytes

The following protocol uses a relatively high collagenase concentration and short digestion time. For higher cell yield, the procedure can be performed in two separate lab sessions by decreasing the collagenase concentration and increasing the digestion time (e.g., 0.018% for 16 h).

1. Prepare the biosafety cabinet (BSC) for use by wiping it down with 70% ethanol and arranging necessary reagents and disposables.
2. Determine the wet weight of the cartilage to be digested:
   a. Measure and record the weight of an empty, sterile petri dish (100 mm diameter or larger).
   b. In the BSC, use sterile forceps to transfer the pieces of cartilage to be digested to the petri dish. Shake off any excess fluid before placing the cartilage into the dish.
   c. Gently aspirate off any remaining liquid surrounding the cartilage, leaving just enough to hydrate the tissue.
   d. Cover the petri dish and re-weigh it to determine the tissue's wet weight.
   e. Immediately rehydrate the tissue with sterile media and set the dish aside in the BSC.
3. Prepare the collagenase solution:
   a. Determine the volume of collagenase solution needed; make 6 mL for every gram of cartilage being digested.
   b. In a 50 mL conical tube, weigh out the appropriate amount of collagenase needed to make a 0.4% solution.
   c. Within the BSC, dissolve the collagenase in chondrocyte media.
   d. Sterilize the collagenase solution by passing it through a 0.2 μm syringe filter. Collect the filtrate in a sterile specimen cup.
   e. Cap the specimen cup and place it in the incubator or 37°C water bath to warm the collagenase solution.
4. Mince the cartilage:
   a. Aspirate off excess media surrounding the cartilage in the petri dish, leaving just enough to maintain tissue hydration.
   b. Carefully mince the cartilage into fragments, each a few cubic millimeters in volume, using a sterile scalpel and forceps.

5. Retrieve the warm collagenase solution, place it in the BSC, and add a sterile stir bar to the specimen cup.

6. Using a sterile spatula, transfer all but a few cartilage fragments into the specimen cup. Keep the "leftover" fragments hydrated because they will be used later to assess cell viability within the tissue.

7. Loosely cap the specimen cup and record the time in your lab notebook. The tissue will be digested in collagenase for 2 h.

8. Lightly spray a magnetic stir plate with 70% ethanol and place it on the bottom shelf of the incubator. Connect the power cord. Place the specimen cup on the stir plate and adjust the speed to stir the solution gently. If it is necessary to run the power cord through the incubator's front door, be sure that the door is closed tightly and the temperature and percentage of CO_2 are stable.

9. While the tissue is digesting, measure the viability of cells within the cartilage:

   a. Transfer two "leftover" cartilage fragments into individual wells of a 96-well plate. It is not necessary to keep the fragments sterile since they will be discarded after viability has been assessed.

   b. With each fragment, mix 2 µL calcein AM, 2 µl EthD-1, and 200 µL PBS.

   c. Cover the plate to protect the samples from light and incubate for 10 min at room temperature. After incubation, the *cytoplasm* of live cells will fluoresce green due to intracellular enzymatic cleavage of the calcein precursor. The *nucleus* of dead cells will fluoresce red because EthD-1 crosses damaged cell membranes and activates after binding to DNA.

   d. *Before* turning on the fluorescent lamp on your microscope, find the filter set(s), also called filter cube(s), that you will be using to visualize the stained tissue. You will use either two separate cubes for visualizing the calcein (EX: 494 nm, EM: 517 nm) and EthD-1 (EX: 494 nm, EM: 517 nm) or one dual emission filter to visualize both dyes simultaneously. The filter cubes are most likely mounted inside a turret on the microscope. Without touching the surface of any filters, note in your lab notebook the manufacturer and product number of the cube(s) that you will be using.

   e. Return the filter cube(s) and turret into their original positions and switch on the fluorescent lamp. Allow the lamp to warm up for ~15 min.

   f. Determine cell viability by counting or estimating the percentage of cells that are alive within a representative region in each cartilage fragment.

   g. Examine multiple regions of the fragments and note any differences in cell viability or staining. Is viability lower near the cut surfaces? Is the whole fragment stained or would a longer incubation time be beneficial?

   h. If a camera is available, capture one or more representative micrographs of the cartilage. Obtain a calibration image so that you will be able to add a scale bar to the micrographs when documenting your results. You may get a calibration image from your instructor or acquire an image of a stage micrometer or hemacytometer grid using the same magnification as in the micrographs.

10. (Optional) Examine the prepared histology slides of hyaline, elastic, and fibrocartilage under a light microscope. In your lab notebook:

    a. Record the stain used to prepare each slide and the source of the tissue.

TABLE 4.1
Guidelines for Initiating Cultures to Obtain a
Density of 100,000 Cells/cm² and to Provide
Sufficient Nutrients between Media Changes

Flask	Culture Area (cm²)	Number of Cells to Inoculate Flask With	Total Media Volume (mL)
T12.5	12.5	1.25×10^6	2.5
T25	25	2.5×10^6	5.0
T75	75	7.5×10^6	15

b. Sketch or describe the arrangement and density of cells within each tissue. Note differences between tissues or in different regions of the same tissue.

c. Describe or sketch the structure and staining of the ECM.

11. At the end of the collagenase incubation period, transfer the specimen cup from the incubator to the BSC and pass the digest through a 40 μm cell strainer into a sterile 50 mL centrifuge tube. The strainer will remove any large, undigested pieces of cartilage from the digest.

12. Wash the chondrocytes by adding 25 mL of 4°C PBS to the conical tube.

13. Spin cells down, using a counterbalance, at 300 g for 5 min and discard the supernatant.

14. Repeat the PBS wash and centrifugation.

15. Resuspend the cell pellet in 1–2 mL of media.

16. Use a hemacytometer and trypan blue to determine the density of cells in the suspension, viability, and total cell yield (refer to hemacytometer protocol in Appendix 2).

17. Plate the cells in one or more tissue culture flasks to achieve a cell density of 100,000 cells/cm² and then add media to reach the total volume indicated in Table 4.1.

18. The chondrocytes can be maintained in culture for 10 days with media changes every 3 days. Longer periods of culture or passaging the cells may lead to dedifferentiation.

4.8 Data Processing and Reporting

Each of the key results to report in text, figure, and/or table format is described next.

1. Report the estimated percentage of viable cells within the tissue and, if applicable, include representative micrographs showing live and dead cells. Summarize your observations related to the homogeneity of cell viability within the cartilage fragments.

2. Include the results of the hemacytometer counts and the calculations used to determine the density of cells in the suspension, viability in the cell suspension, and total cell yield.

3. Report the total wet weight of the cartilage that was digested and the number of viable cells isolated per gram of tissue. Compare your results and methods with those reported in the literature by other investigators who have isolated chondrocytes from calf articular cartilage. Cite your sources.

4. Calculate the *efficiency* of the isolation protocol. Assume that the cartilage contained exactly 50×10^6 cells per gram wet weight (Kim et al. 1988). Use the percentage viability measured in the LIVE/DEAD assay and measured wet weight to estimate the number of viable cells originally within the cartilage.

4.9 Prelab Questions

1. From the media recipe, calculate the concentration of l-proline and l-glutamine in chondrocyte media. *Note: Do not include the l-proline present in the nonessential amino acid solution in your calculation.*

2. The concentration of collagenase used to isolate the chondrocytes is expressed as a percentage. Two alternate methods of expressing enzyme concentration are weight per volume (e.g., milligrams per milliliter) and units of enzyme activity per volume (e.g., units per milliliter). Conversion between percentage and weight is straightforward using the definition of a 1% solution, 1 g of solute in 100 mL of solvent. Conversion to units of activity per volume is more complicated because, while percentage and weight per volume are based on physical characteristics that are easily determined, a unit of activity is a measure of the biochemical function of the enzyme. As such, a unit of activity per gram varies for different types of collagenase or different lots of the same collagenase and can easily change over time. Furthermore, a "unit" of activity is often defined differently by different investigators (McCarthy et al. 2011).

   a. Express the enzyme concentration used in the isolation protocol in milligrams per milliliter.

   b. What is the approximate activity of the collagenase reported on the product data sheet for the collagenase that you will use? Briefly describe how the activity was measured, including the temperature, pH, and substrate used in the activity assay. Cite your sources.

   c. Approximate the enzyme concentration used in the isolation protocol in units per milliliter.

   d. Is one method better for reporting enzyme concentration? Justify your answer.

3. Freshly isolated cartilage can be stored at 4°C for 14 days or 37°C for 28 days with minimal loss of cell viability (Williams et al. 2003; Pallante et al. 2009). What properties of cartilage lead to the tissue's survivability outside the body? Briefly explain your answer.

4. The density of chondrocytes cultured in monolayer influences their phenotype. At low densities (e.g., 10,000 cells/cm²), chondrocytes have a tendency to lose their specific differentiated phenotype; they are more stable when cultured at a high density (e.g., ≥100,000 cells/cm²) (von der Mark et al. 1977). To establish a high-density culture, the final step of this lab involves inoculating a tissue culture flask with a specific number of cells. Assume that after resuspending the cells in media, diluting 40 μL of the cell suspension with 10 μL trypan blue, as described in Appendix 2, and loading two samples on the hemacytometer, you count 100 and 105 cells in the central 25 squares. Calculate the volume of the cell suspension that should be added to a T25 flask to achieve a density of 100,000 cells/cm². Show your work.

5. During this experiment, chondrocytes are removed from the collagenase solution and rinsed using centrifugation. Lab centrifuges have either a *fixed* or *swinging bucket* rotor. With a swinging bucket rotor, centrifuge tubes are placed into tube holders, or

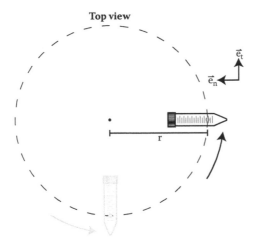

Figure 4.3
Top view of a conical tube rotating in a horizontal, circular path as it would in a centrifuge with a swinging bucket rotor. The distance between the axis of rotation and a representative cell within the tube is r. The unit vectors, $\vec{e}_n$ and $\vec{e}_t$, are in the directions tangential and normal to the cell's path at the instant shown.

"buckets," that are attached to the rotor by hinges. As the rotor turns, the buckets swing out, the sample rotates in a horizontal plane around the center axis, and the precipitant (e.g., cells) is driven to the bottom of the centrifuge tube (Figure 4.3).

a. The total acceleration of a cell traveling a circular path of radius (r) within a centrifuge can be written in terms of components that are normal ($\vec{e}_n$) and tangential ($\vec{e}_t$) to the cell's path:

$$\vec{a} = \vec{a}_t + \vec{a}_n \tag{4.1}$$

$$\vec{a} = \frac{dv}{dt}\vec{e}_t + \frac{v^2}{r}\vec{e}_n \tag{4.2}$$

The tangential component of the acceleration is 0 for a cell traveling the path at a constant velocity $= v$; therefore,

$$\vec{a} = \frac{v^2}{r}\vec{e}_n \tag{4.3}$$

Use the preceding equation and Newton's second law to derive an expression for relative centrifugal force (RCF) in terms of r and revolutions per minute (RPM). *Hint: the force exerted on the cell is traditionally expressed **relative** to the force exerted due to gravity (mg)—specifically, RCF × mg.*

b. Use information supplied by the manufacturer of the centrifuge you will be using or measure the average radius of curvature. Determine how many RPMs corresponds to an RCF of 300 g.

TABLE 4.2

Sample Data from a Spectrophotometric Assay to Determine the Activity of a Collagenase Solution

Time (min)	A_{320nm}
0	0
5	0.5
10	1.35
15	1.7
20	2.39

6. Table 4.2 shows data obtained from an assay to measure the activity of a collagenase solution similar to the solution used to digest cartilage in this lab. The assay is based on the increase in absorbance at 320 nm that occurs when collagenase cleaves a synthetic peptide into two smaller fragments. To obtain the data, 20 μL of the collagenase solution is added to a cuvette containing 980 μL of the synthetic peptide in a buffer at 25°C and pH 7.1. The absorbance of the cuvette, relative to a cuvette containing the synthetic peptide but no collagenase, was measured at 0, 5, 10, 15, and 20 min. The molar extinction coefficient, ε, is a measure of the amount of light of a particular wavelength absorbed by a substance. It depends on concentration and the distance the light must travel through the substance according to the Beer–Lambert law: $A = \varepsilon C l$, where A is the absorbance (unitless) at the wavelength of interest, C is the concentration of the substrate (mol/length³), and l is the path length (length) equal to 1 cm for a standard cuvette. It is evident from the equation that ε has dimensions of (length²/mol). In this experiment, the extinction coefficient of the fragments produced by collagenase digestion is 21 cm²/μmol.

a. Plot the preceding data and use linear regression to determine the change in absorbance with time.

b. Calculate the activity of the original enzyme solution in units per milliliter. For this assay, a unit is defined as the amount of enzyme needed to liberate 1 μmol of the fragments in 1 min at 25°C and pH 7.1. *Hint: use dimensional analysis and your understanding of the experiment to determine the appropriate equation.*

4.10 Postlab Questions

1. Bovine calf cartilage contains ~50 × 10⁶ cells per gram wet weight of tissue (Kim et al. 1988).

a. Use the calculated cell yield (cells per milligram wet weight) and percentage viability measured in the LIVE/DEAD assay to estimate the *apparent* density of chondrocytes within the tissue from which the cells were isolated. Show your calculations.

b. The density calculated in part *a* is likely less than the reported value of ~50 × 10⁶ cells per gram wet weight. List as many possible reasons for this discrepancy as you can think of.

2. In the Carticel procedure, a surgeon must collect two small biopsies of the patient's cartilage from which the chondrocytes are isolated and subsequently expanded in culture. The recommended size of each biopsy is 5 mm × 8 mm × the full thickness of the cartilage.

   a. Estimate the total number of cells in the two biopsies, assuming the patient's cartilage is 3 mm thick, the density of cells within the tissue is 10×10^6 cells per gram wet weight, and the density of cartilage is approximately equal to that of water. Show your calculations.

   b. Each patient is supplied with at least 12 million cells for implantation into his or her cartilage defect. Based on the calculation in part (a), determine the minimum number of cell divisions that the chondrocytes must undergo to yield 12 million cells. Show your calculations.

   c. The calculation in part (b) assumes that 100% of the native cells are successfully isolated from the cartilage biopsies. If the efficiency of cell isolation was similar to what you achieved in this lab, how many cell divisions would the isolated chondrocytes need to undergo to yield 12 million cells?

3. Chondrocytes cultured in monolayer under a variety of conditions have been shown to lose their specific differentiated phenotype, characterized by the production of type II collagen. Design and briefly describe an experiment that could be used to determine how long the cells you isolated continue to express the chondrocyte phenotype. Cite your references.

4. As part of data processing, you calculated the efficiency of cell isolation using the assumption that the cartilage contained exactly 50×10^6 cells per gram wet weight. Describe a method that could be used directly to measure cartilage cellularity to give a more accurate measure of efficiency compared to using an average value found in the literature.

5. The manufacturer and product number of the filter cube or cubes used to visualize the LIVE/DEAD dyes were recorded during the experiment.

   a. Visit the manufacturer's website to find the specifications of each filter cube used and sketch the transmission spectrum of the excitation filter, dichroic mirror, and emission filter. Indicate the *maximum* excitation and emission wavelength for the dyes in the LIVE/DEAD assay on the graph(s).

   b. Briefly describe the path of the light as it moved from the fluorescent lamp through the filters, to the sample, and eventually to your eye. Be specific with respect to which wavelengths pass through each filter and which are reflected. *Note: Fluorescent dyes typically excite over a range of wavelengths near the maximum excitation wavelength.*

References

Brittberg, M., A. Lindahl, A. Nilsson, C. Ohlsson, O. Isaksson, and L. Peterson. 1994. Treatment of deep cartilage defects in the knee with autologous chondrocyte transplantation. *New England Journal of Medicine* 331 (14): 889–895.

Freeman, M. A. 1979. *Adult articular cartilage.* Philadelphia: J. B. Lippincott Co.

Freshney, R. I. 2010. *Culture of animal cells: A manual of basic technique and specialized applications.* New York: John Wiley & Sons.

Genzyme Corporation. 2011. Treatment with Carticel. Available from http://www.carticel. com/patients/treatment.aspx (accessed July 2011).

Hunziker, E., M. Spector, J. Libera, A. Gertzman, S. L. Woo, A. Ratcliffe, M. Lysaght, A. Coury, D. Kaplan, and G. Vunjak-Novakovic. 2006. Translation from research to applications. *Tissue Engineering* 12 (12): 3341–3364.

Kim, Y. J., R. L. Sah, J. Y. Doong, and A. J. Grodzinsky. 1988. Fluorometric assay of DNA in cartilage explants using Hoechst 33258. *Analytical Biochemistry* 174 (1): 168–176.

McCarthy, R. C., A. G. Breite, M. L. Green, and F. E. Dwulet. 2011. Tissue dissociation enzymes for isolating human islets for transplantation: Factors to consider in setting enzyme acceptance criteria. *Transplantation* 91 (2): 137–145.

Minas, T., and L. Peterson. 2006. *Surgical manual for the implantation of cultured autologous chondrocytes*. Cambridge, MA: Genzyme Biosurgery.

Molecular Probes. 2005. LIVE/DEAD viability/cytotoxicity kit. Available from http://tools. invitrogen.com/content/sfs/manuals/mp03224.pdf (accessed January 2012).

Pallante, A. L., W. C. Bae, A. C. Chen, S. Gortz, W. D. Bugbee, and R. L. Sah. 2009. Chondrocyte viability is higher after prolonged storage at 37 degrees C than at 4 degrees C for osteochondral grafts. *American Journal of Sports Medicine* 37 Suppl 1: 24S–32S.

von der Mark, K., V. Gauss, H. von der Mark, and P. Muller. 1977. Relationship between cell shape and type of collagen synthesized as chondrocytes lose their cartilage phenotype in culture. *Nature* 267 (5611): 531–532.

Williams, S. K., D. Amiel, S. T. Ball, R. T. Allen, V. W. Wong, A. C. Chen, R. L. Sah, and W. D. Bugbee. 2003. Prolonged storage effects on the articular cartilage of fresh human osteochondral allografts. *Journal of Bone and Joint Surgery* (American vol. 85-A) (11): 2111–2120.

Wood, J. J., M. A. Malek, F. J. Frassica, J. A. Polder, A. K. Mohan, E. T. Bloom, M. M. Braun, and T. R. Cote. 2006. Autologous cultured chondrocytes: Adverse events reported to the United States Food and Drug Administration. *Journal of Bone and Joint Surgery* (American vol. 88) (3): 503–507.

Zaslav, K., B. Cole, R. Brewster, T. DeBerardino, J. Farr, P. Fowler, and C. Nissen. 2009. A prospective study of autologous chondrocyte implantation in patients with failed prior treatment for articular cartilage defect of the knee: Results of the Study of the Treatment of Articular Repair (STAR) clinical trial. *American Journal of Sports Medicine* 37 (1): 42–55.

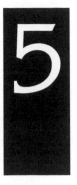

Chapter 5

Measuring and Modeling Growth of a Cell Population

5.1 Background

Cell-based tissue-engineering therapies typically require tens of millions to billions of cells per patient. In general, it is not feasible to isolate sufficient quantities of primary cells directly from tissue. To expand the number available, cells are cultured in conditions that stimulate cell division.

Adherent cells can be expanded in number by plating, or seeding, a culture dish with a low density of cells (Figure 5.1a) and then maintaining the culture to allow the cells to attach (Figure 5.1b) and proliferate enough to nearly cover the culture surface (Figure 5.1c). When the cells cover the entire culture surface, the culture is said to be confluent. Once a monolayer culture is *nearly* confluent, cells are dissociated from the surface and neighboring cells using the proteolytic enzyme trypsin and replated at a lower density in multiple culture dishes (Figure 5.1d). The process of transferring cells from one culture vessel to another to allow further growth is called *subculturing* or *passaging*. By subculturing primary cells, an *early passage cell line* is established (Freshney 2010).

The process of subculturing may cause some cells to lose important phenotype-specific behaviors—namely, to dedifferentiate. Altering culture conditions such as the media formulation, substrate protein coating, or geometry may slow or reverse the dedifferentiation process. Culture conditions may also be modified to favor proliferation of a single cell type within a heterogeneous cell population, such as is typical in a primary culture. By stimulating proliferation of one cell type more than others it is possible to increase the proportion of cells that are the cell type of interest, thus enriching the population.

A normal cell population cannot be expanded infinitely because the number of cell divisions a single cell can undergo in culture is limited. The Hayflick limit predicts that normal cells in culture can divide a maximum of 50 times under optimal conditions before they cease dividing or become senescent (Rubin 2002). Some cell lines may become immortalized through spontaneous or induced genetic mutation (Freshney 2010). These immortalized cell lines are experimentally convenient

53

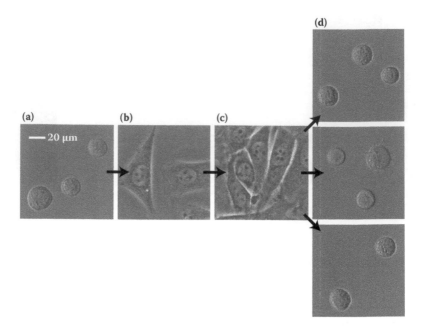

Figure 5.1
Time course of fibroblasts growing in a monolayer culture. (a) Immediately after seeding, cells appear round under the microscope because they have not attached to the culture surface. (b) Within a day, cells attach and spread. (c) The density of cells on the culture surface increases as the cells proliferate. (d) When the cells are nearly confluent, they are trypsinized and plated at a low density into several culture vessels to continue expanding the cells in number.

because of their ability to divide without limit; however, they are fundamentally different from the normal population of cells from which they were derived. Some of the most commonly used cell lines are 3T3 (mouse fibroblasts), HeLa (human epithelial cells), CHO (Chinese hamster ovary cells), H1 (human embryonic stem cells), and C2C12 (mouse myoblasts).

Cell growth in culture can be monitored by plotting the density (or number) of cells versus time in culture. Multiple experimental methods can be used to measure the number of cells in culture at a particular point in time. The most common method involves releasing cells from culture and counting a representative volume of the suspension using a hemacytometer or Coulter Counter®. In this experiment, you will collect data to construct a growth curve using a commercially available fluorescence-based DNA assay called PicoGreen®.

A typical growth curve is plotted on a semilog scale and has three distinct phases: lag, exponential growth, and plateau (Figure 5.2) (Vunjak-Novakovic and Freshney 2006; Freshney 2010). The first 12–24 h after initiating a culture is typically a period of negligible proliferation. This lag phase represents the time required for cells to recover from isolation, thawing, or passaging and then to attach firmly to the culture surface and to reenter the cell cycle. After the lag phase, cells begin to double at a regular interval, called the doubling time (t_d), and growth is exponential.

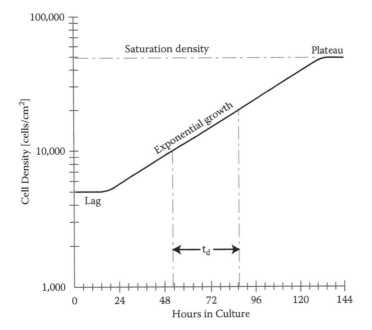

Figure 5.2
Representative growth curve showing lag, exponential growth, and plateau phases. The doubling time (t_d) can be determined during the exponential growth phase by measuring the interval over which the population doubles in size. The saturation density is the maximum cell density achieved before the cells stop proliferating due to contact inhibition or nutrient limitations.

The doubling time varies depending on cell type and culture conditions from a minimum of 12 h to essentially infinity because some cell types do not proliferate in culture (Palsson and Bhatia 2004). At the end of the exponential growth phase, the cell monolayer is dense and proliferation is inhibited by contact with neighboring cells. As a result, the growth curve reaches the plateau phase. The maximum density at the plateau phase is called the saturation density.

Mathematical models can be used to describe and predict cell growth in culture. In the early stages of culture, growth is unconstrained and the rate of increase in cell number (dX/dt) is approximately proportional to the number of cells currently in culture (X):

$$\frac{dX}{dt} \propto X \tag{5.1}$$

Defining the growth rate, μ, as the proportionality constant and integrating with X_0 as the initial number of cells in culture gives the exponential growth equation:

$$\frac{dX}{dt} = \mu X \tag{5.2}$$

$$\int_{X_0}^{X} \frac{1}{X} dX = \mu \int_{0}^{t} dt \qquad (5.3)$$

$$\ln \frac{X}{X_0} = \mu t \qquad (5.4)$$

$$X = X_0 e^{\mu t} \qquad (5.5)$$

An equivalent equation can be written in terms of doubling time (t_d) rather than growth rate (μ):

$$X = X_0 2^{t/t_d} \qquad (5.6)$$

The relationship between μ and t_d can be found:

$$\frac{X}{X_0} = e^{\mu t} \qquad (5.7)$$

$$2 = e^{\mu t_d} \qquad (5.8)$$

$$\frac{\ln 2}{\mu} = t_d \qquad (5.9)$$

In reality, cells in a culture vessel do not grow without limit due to space and/or nutrient constraints. To model constrained growth, a term can be added to Equation 5.2 that will decrease the rate of creation of new cells as the number of cells in culture reaches saturation (X_{max}). Specifically,

$$\frac{dX}{dt} = \mu X \left(1 - \frac{X}{X_{max}} \right) \qquad (5.10)$$

Note that when X is very small, the effect of this term is negligible but, as X approaches X_{max}, the effect is dominant. The solution to the constrained growth equation is

$$X = \frac{X_0}{X_0/X_{max} + \left[1 - \left(X_0/X_{max} \right) \right] e^{-\mu t}} \qquad (5.11)$$

The preceding models can be used to compare culture conditions quantitatively to determine which conditions optimize cell growth and to determine the appropriate interval to passage cells. Having an efficient and reliable protocol for generating large quantities of cells is essential for scaling up experimental cell-based tissue-engineering therapies for commercialization.

5.2 Learning Objectives

The objectives of this experiment are to

- Master essential lab skills including sterile technique, changing media, trypsinization, and cell counting using a hemacytometer
- Learn to perform a widely applicable DNA assay using a fluorometer
- Monitor cell growth to determine the effect of serum concentration on cell proliferation and to distinguish the phases of growth: lag, exponential, and plateau
- Fit experimental data to a mathematical model of constrained growth to estimate the growth rate for each media formulation
- Compare cell counts obtained using a hemacytometer to those obtained from the fluorescence-based DNA assay

5.3 Overview of Experiment

In this experiment, you will characterize the kinetics of cell growth and investigate the effect of serum concentration on growth rate. In the first lab session, monolayer cultures will be established in media supplemented with 5%, 10%, or 20% serum. Each day thereafter for 1 week (sessions 2–8), a subset of the cultures will be terminated to later measure the number of cells in the culture using PicoGreen, a fluorescence DNA-binding dye (Figure 5.3). Your instructor may terminate some of the samples for you or may specify that samples should be terminated only on specific weekdays.

At one or more time points, additional samples will be collected by trypsinizing the cells and counting them using a hemacytometer. Data from the PicoGreen assay and the hemacytometer counts will be compared. Consult your instructor to determine which days you should perform the hemacytometer counts. The PicoGreen assay will be run in the last session after all the samples have been collected. The experimental data will be fit to a mathematical model of constrained growth and used to calculate a growth rate for cells in each media formulation.

5.4 Safety Notes

According to the manufacturer, the mutagenicity and toxicity of PicoGreen have not been assessed. Because this reagent binds to nucleic acids, it should be treated

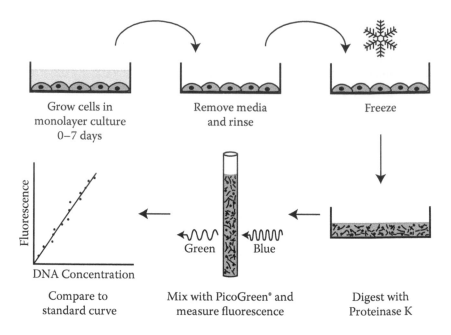

Figure 5.3
Overview of the procedure that will be used to track the number of cells in culture over time. Populations of cells are grown in monolayer culture. At various time points, samples are collected and frozen until the last day of the experiment. At that time, the cell monolayers are enzymatically digested, the digest is stained with the DNA-binding dye, and the resulting fluorescence measured using a fluorometer. A standard curve, generated from samples with known DNA concentrations, is used to convert fluorescence of the sample to number of cells in culture.

as a potential mutagen, handled with care, and disposed of in accordance with local regulations. Use good lab practices and review all relevant MSDSs.

5.5 Materials

In addition to the general equipment and supplies, the following are needed to complete this experiment:

5.5.1 Reagents and Consumables

- ~2×10^6 3T3 Cells in culture (e.g., 1×100 mm confluent dish)
- DMEM
- Bovine calf serum (BCS)
- 100X Penicillin/streptomycin (P/S)
- 0.25% Trypsin with EDTA (1X)
- Trypan blue

- 48-Well tissue-culture-treated plates
- 1X Phosphate-buffered saline (PBS)
- Phosphate-buffered EDTA (PBE)
- 50X Proteinase-K (25 mg/mL in PBE)
- PicoGreen dsDNA assay kit (including TE buffer and 100 µg/mL DNA standard; Molecular Probes)

5.5.2 Equipment and Supplies

- Promega Quanti-Fluor fluorometer (EX: 480 nm, EM: 520 nm) with minicell cuvettes (a plate reader can be used instead of a fluorometer if one is available)
- Water bath (with rack to position samples above water)

5.6 Recipes

1X PBS. Add 50 mL 10X PBS (with Ca^{2+} and Mg^{2+}) to 400 mL deionized H_2O (dH_2O). Mix well, adjust pH to 7.4 with HCl and NaOH, bring total volume to 500 mL with dH_2O, and either sterile-filter through a 0.2 µm filter or autoclave.

0.1 M Phosphate buffer. Reconstitute according to manufacturer's instructions or purchase 1X solution.

PBE. Dissolve ethylenediaminetetraacetic acid disodium salt dihydrate (EDTA, MW = 372) at 1.86 mg/mL in 0.1 M phosphate buffer, adjust pH to 7.1 with HCl and NaOH, and store at room temperature (RT).

50X Proteinase-K stock. Dilute proteinase-K in PBE to a concentration of 25 mg/mL, prepare 100 µL aliquots, and store at –20°C for up to a year. This is a 50X stock solution. Dilute the stock in PBE as needed.

1X TE buffer. Dilute the 20X TE buffer supplied with the PicoGreen kit in dH_2O.

100 µg/mL DNA standard. Prepare 5 µL aliquots of the DNA standard provided with the PicoGreen kit. Store at –20°C.

PicoGreen. Prepare 5 µL aliquots of the 200X solution provided with the PicoGreen kit. Store at –20°C.

5.7 Methods

5.7.1 Session 1: Initiate the Cell Cultures

1. Thaw ~10 mL of BCS, 5 mL of 100X P/S, and ~4 mL of trypsin in a 37°C water bath.
2. Prepare the biosafety cabinet (BSC) for use by wiping it down with 70% ethanol and arranging necessary reagents and disposables.
3. Make the media formulations:

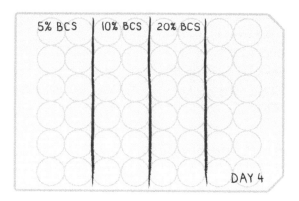

Figure 5.4
Label one 48-well plate for each day that the number of cells in culture will be measured. Arrange the samples within the 48-well plate and label the lid as shown here.

    a. In the BSC, add 5 mL of the P/S to a 500 mL bottle of DMEM.

    b. In three separate conical tubes, make 35 mL of DMEM + 5% BCS and 15 mL each of DMEM + 10% and DMEM + 20% BCS. Warm the media to 37°C in the water bath or incubator.

    c. For each day that the cells will be assayed, label the lid of one 48-well plate as shown in Figure 5.4. For example, you will need seven separate plates if you plan to measure the number of cells in culture every day for 1 week. The day that the cultures are initiated is "day 0," the next day is "day 1," and so on. Do not prepare a plate for day 0.

4. Prepare the cell suspension:

    a. Remove the dish or flask of cells you have been given from the incubator.

    b. Observe the cells using phase contrast microscopy. Document the extent of confluence and cell morphology in your lab notebook.

    c. Trypsinize the cells (refer to trypsinization protocol in Appendix 1), rinse once in DMEM + 5% BCS, spin down, and discard the supernatant.

    d. Resuspend the cells in 1 mL of DMEM + 5% BCS.

    e. Count the cells using a hemacytometer (refer to hemacytometer protocol in Appendix 2).

    f. Dilute the suspension to a final concentration of 0.5×10^6 cells/mL in DMEM + 5% BCS.

    g. In three new conical tubes, combine 250 μL of the well-mixed cell suspension with 4.75 mL DMEM + 5%, DMEM + 10%, or DMEM + 20% BCS to achieve a final cell concentration of 25,000 cells/mL. Store extra medium in the refrigerator so that it can be used for future media changes.

    h. Save 200 μL of each cell suspension in individual vials with threaded caps (e.g., cryovial). Label the vials and store them in a −20°C freezer until the final day of the experiment.

5. For each sample, add 200 μL of the appropriate cell suspension to a single well in a 48-well plate. For the PicoGreen assay, prepare two samples per serum concentration

per day ($n = 2$). For the specific days where you will also perform manual counts with the hemacytometer, prepare two additional samples per serum concentration ($n = 2$). Remember to periodically mix the cell suspensions and to use a different plate for each day the cells will be assayed.

6. Note the time at which the cultures were initiated in your lab notebook.

7. Place the plates in the incubator.

8. If time permits, wait ~30 min and then observe several wells under the microscope to verify that the desired cell density was approximately achieved and that the cells are beginning to attach to the culture-treated plastic surface.

9. Maintain the cultures in the incubator, change media every third day, and collect samples daily as described in Section 5.7.2.

5.7.2 Sessions 2–8: Terminate the Cultures

Every day (or as often as possible), one plate of cultures should be terminated and samples collected for the PicoGreen assay (see following step 1 and Appendix 3). At one or more time points, trypsinize parallel samples and perform manual counts with the hemacytometer so that the counts can be compared (see step 2). Warm ~1 mL of trypsin in a 37°C water bath before beginning the lab if you plan to trypsinize cells for hemacytometer counting.

1. Collect samples for the PicoGreen assay:

   a. Remove one multiwell culture plate from the incubator.

   b. Observe the cells using phase contrast microscopy. In your lab notebook, record the time and document the extent of confluence, cell morphology, and variability that exists in the distribution of cells within the well.

   c. Aspirate the media from each well.

   d. Rinse each well once with 200 μL of PBS and aspirate to remove the rinse.

   e. If you are trypsinizing samples for hemacytometer counting, add 200 μL of PBS to just those wells and proceed to step 2. If not, freeze the plate at −80°C (or −20°C) until all the samples have been collected and you are ready to perform the PicoGreen assay.

2. Collect samples for hemacytometer counting:

   a. In the BSC, pipette ~2 mL of DMEM + 10% BCS into a conical tube. Return the bottle of media to the refrigerator. *Note: All other steps in this procedure can be performed outside the BSC.*

   b. Aspirate the PBS from each sample that you plan to count with the hemacytometer and replace with 100 μL of warmed trypsin (there should be two samples per serum concentration). Gently swirl the plate to cover the entire well with trypsin.

   c. Wait for the cells to detach and then add 150 μL of DMEM + 10% BCS. Pipette up and down a few times to detach all the cells and to generate a uniform cell suspension.

   d. Working quickly but carefully, count a portion of each cell suspension on the hemacytometer. *Note: The density of cells on the hemacytometer may be low depending on how many days the cells have been in culture. If so, count multiple fields and average them so that you have a reasonable estimate of the true cell density.*

e. Calculate the number of cells present in the well prior to trypsinization. Record the raw hemacytometer counts and these calculations in your lab notebook.

f. Aspirate the trypsin-media mixture from the wells and discard.

g. Freeze the plate at –80°C (or –20°C) until all the samples have been collected and you are ready to perform the PicoGreen assay.

5.7.3 Final Session: Perform the PicoGreen® Assay

1. Warm a water bath to 50°C.

2. Remove the multiwell plates, one proteinase-K aliquot, PicoGreen dye (one 5 µL aliquot per mL of dye needed; see Appendix 3), DNA standards, and the cell suspension samples collected from the freezer during Session 1.

3. Make a 0.5 mg/mL proteinase-K solution by combining 100 µL of the 50X (25 mg/mL) stock solution with 4.9 mL PBE.

4. Add 100 µL of proteinase-K to each well of the plates that contains cells to be measured. Cover and stack the plates and place them in a 50°C water bath on a rack above the water level. Make sure that the plates are flat so that the entire cell monolayer is covered with proteinase-K. Add 200 µL proteinase-K to each cryovial containing a sample of the cell suspension and place them in the water bath, also above the water level. Place the cover over the water bath.

5. Incubate for ≥30 min at 50°C. While waiting, prepare and measure the DNA standards:

   a. Turn on and configure the fluorometer to excite at ~480 nm and measure emission at ~520 nm.

   b. Prepare the PicoGreen dye solution as described in the PicoGreen protocol (Appendix 3).

   c. Prepare the DNA standards (200–0 ng DNA/mL final volume) as described in the PicoGreen protocol.

   d. Generate a standard curve as described in the PicoGreen protocol. If the standard curve is not linear, try to identify the source of error and repeat until a reliable standard curve is obtained.

6. After the plates have incubated for ≥30 min, use a microscope to verify that the cell monolayer has released off the bottom of the plates. Homogenize the samples by pipetting up and down *vigorously*.

7. Prepare duplicate samples for the DNA assay. It is easiest to dilute the samples in empty wells within the same plate. For this particular experiment, mixing 10 µL of each sample with 190 µL TE buffer should yield a concentration within the range of the standards. *Note: It is very important to mix each sample thoroughly before and after diluting it.*

8. Perform the PicoGreen assay to measure the DNA concentration in each sample. If any sample is out of range of the standards or the fluorometer detection limit, dilute

the sample more and repeat the measurement until the reading falls within the working range of the calibration curve. Make careful notes regarding the dilutions in your lab notebook.

5.8 Data Processing and Reporting

Briefly report the results of your experiment in paragraph and graphical form. Each of the key results to report in text, figure, and/or table format is described next.

1. Include a graph of the DNA standard curve (x-axis: DNA concentration; y-axis: fluorescence). Display the equation of the standard curve and the r^2 value on the graph.

2. Include a table, similar to Table 5.1, displaying the raw fluorescence data and corresponding cell number measured using the PicoGreen assay. Briefly describe any necessary calculations in the text. *Note: The DNA content of a 3T3 cell is 13.7 pg/cell* (Patterson 1979).

3. Report the average saturation density (X_{max}), in cells per square centimeter, for each media formulation. Comment on whether saturation density appears to depend appreciably on serum concentration.

4. Use the equation for constrained growth (Equation 5.10) to calculate the growth rate for cells in each of the media formulations. This can be accomplished by rearranging

TABLE 5.1
Suggested Format for Reporting Data Collected from the DNA Assay

	Sample Description						
	Day 0 (Cell Suspension)			Day 1			Day 2
	5%	10%	20%	5%	10%	20%	5%...
Fluorescence							
Fluorescence of duplicate							
Mean fluorescence							
Percentage difference in duplicates							
[DNA] in cuvette[a] (picograms/milliliter)							
Dilution factor[b]							
[DNA] in sample (picograms/milliliter)							
[Cells] in sample (cells/milliliter)							
Total cells in sample							

[a] Calculate from the average fluorescence and the standard curve.
[b] Dilution factor = total volume in cuvette ÷ volume of undiluted sample in cuvette.

the constrained growth equation such that the growth rate is the slope of the best fit line relating time to some function of X_0, X, and X_{max}. Briefly summarize the calculations performed and include a graph of the curve fit.

5. Generate a graph of the experimental data displaying population growth with time for the different media formulations (x-axis: time in culture; y-axis: number of cells in culture). Superimpose on the experimental data the predictions of the constrained growth model using the growth rate calculated previously. Discuss how well the model fits the experimental data and suggest possible reasons for discrepancies.

6. Report on the agreement or disagreement of the manual cell counts from the hemacytometer and the data from the PicoGreen assay. For both types of measurements, quantify the variability and discuss possible sources of error.

5.9 Prelab Questions

1. Calculate the planned initial density (X_0) of the cells within the 48-well plate. Report your answer as cells/cm^2.

2. This experiment tests the hypothesis that growth rate, under the conditions used here, depends on serum concentration in the media. What class of proteins is found in serum that may result in different growth rates being observed?

3. Assume you have a population of cells that grows exponentially when subconfluent and has a doubling time of 18 h. If you recover 7×10^6 cells from a T75 flask that was 80% confluent and split the cells 1:8, how long would it take for the passaged cells to reach 80% confluence? Show your calculations.

4. Show that the two expressions given for unconstrained growth in the introduction,

$$X = X_0 e^{\mu t} \quad \text{and} \quad X = X_0 2^{t/t_d}$$

are equivalent.

5. Each standard and sample is measured in duplicate for the PicoGreen assay. If the duplicate measures are similar, does that indicate high precision or high accuracy in the measurement? Briefly explain.

6. In this experiment, a suspension of 25,000 cells/mL is made by mixing 250 μL of a 500,000 cells/mL suspension with 4.75 mL of media. Calculate the percentage error in the final cell density associated with each of the following scenarios. In each case, assume the worst case scenario (maximum error occurs when the cell suspension volume is higher than the desired volume and the media volume is lower):

   a. The concentrated cell suspension is measured using a 1 mL serological pipette with an accuracy of ±10 μL. The media are measured using a 5 mL serological pipette with an accuracy of ±100 μL.

   b. The concentrated cell suspension is measured using a 1000 μL micropipette, which has an accuracy of ±3 μL when dispensing 250 μL. The media are measured using a 5 mL serological pipette, which has an accuracy of ±100 μL.

   c. The concentrated cell suspension is measured using a 1000 μL micropipette, which has an accuracy of ±3 μL when dispensing 250 μL. The media are measured by repeated pipetting using a 1000 μL micropipette, which has an accuracy of ±8 μL when dispensing 950 μL.

d. Briefly discuss the results of your calculations.

5.10 Postlab Questions

1. An accurate growth model is useful for developing standard operating procedures for routine cell maintenance or manufacturing:

    a. Determine the initial seeding density required if you want to passage cells, at 80% confluence, every 72 h. Use the measured growth rate and saturation density from the cultures in 10% serum.

    b. Repeat the calculation using an unconstrained growth model with the growth rate and saturation density in (a). Are the answers substantially different? Why or why not?

2. The plateau phase of growth should be evident in your data. Briefly describe a follow-up experiment that could be conducted to test whether cell proliferation slowed due to limitation in nutrients or space.

3. Briefly describe two alternative methods that could have been used to determine the number of cells in culture over time. Cite your references, if any.

4. Calculate the doubling time corresponding to the growth rate you observed for the cultures in 10% serum. Compare this experimentally observed doubling time with that reported on the product data sheet or in the literature for 3T3 cells.

References

Freshney, R. I. 2010. *Culture of animal cells: A manual of basic technique and specialized applications.* New York: John Wiley & Sons.

Palsson, B. O., and S. N. Bhatia. 2004. *Tissue engineering.* Upper Saddle River, NJ: Pearson Education.

Patterson, M. K., Jr. 1979. Measurement of growth and viability of cells in culture. In *Methods in enzymology,* ed. I. H. P. William B. Jakoby. New York: Academic Press.

Rubin, H. 2002. The disparity between human cell senescence in vitro and lifelong replication in vivo. *Nature Biotechnology* 20 (7): 675–681.

Vunjak-Novakovic, G., and R. I. Freshney. 2006. *Culture of cells for tissue engineering.* Hoboken, NJ: John Wiley & Sons.

Purification of a Cell Population Using Magnetic Cell Sorting

6.1 Background

The adult human body contains more than 200 different cell types, organized in complex combinations with extracellular matrix components to form tissues (Alberts et al. 2007). For tissue-engineering applications, it is often necessary to isolate one cell type from a heterogeneous population acquired from a tissue biopsy or dissection. For example, adult stem cells can be isolated from a human bone marrow biopsy but there are 10^4 "contaminating" cells for every one stem cell (Lin and Goodell 2011). Cells of interest, also called *target* cells, are routinely isolated from a heterogeneous population based on physical properties, the ability to adhere to a substrate, or the presence of specific cell surface receptors.

The most common method for separating cells based on physical properties is centrifugation. In *differential* centrifugation, cells are suspended in a homogeneous solution and centrifuged, causing cells to sediment at different rates based on their size and density. If the cells are assumed to be a perfect sphere in a Newtonian fluid, the sedimentation velocity (V) can be calculated from a balance of forces acting on the cell, including the buoyancy force, gravitational force, and drag force:

$$V = \frac{2r^2}{9\mu}(\rho_c - \rho_f)g \qquad (6.1)$$

where
r is the cell radius
μ is the fluid viscosity
ρ_c and ρ_f are the densities of the cell and fluid, respectively
g is the centrifugal acceleration

In *density gradient* centrifugation, a cell suspension is added to the top of a tube filled with a solution varying from low density at the top to high density at the bottom

(Figure 6.1a). As the sample is centrifuged, bands of cells with similar sedimentation rates form. Differential and density gradient centrifugation can be used to separate cells in bulk, however, with relatively low purity.

Another method for bulk cell sorting is based on preferential adhesion to a culture substrate (Figure 6.1b). A mixed population of cells is seeded onto a tissue-culture-treated or protein-coated dish and the cells are allowed to attach for a short period of time (minutes to hours) before the nonadherent cells are removed with the media. Separation based on preferential adhesion is easy and convenient and has been used to purify adipose-derived stem cells from lipoaspirates (Zuk et al. 2001). This method is limited, however, in that it can only be used to separate cell populations with intrinsically different adhesive properties and the resulting population is not as pure as can be achieved using methods based on specific cell surface receptors, as described next.

Phenotypically different cells perform different functions in the body and, consequently, express different receptors on their cell membrane. Cell-surface receptors that are characteristic of a specific cell phenotype, called *markers*, can be used to isolate those cells from a heterogeneous population. Specifically, the heterogeneous

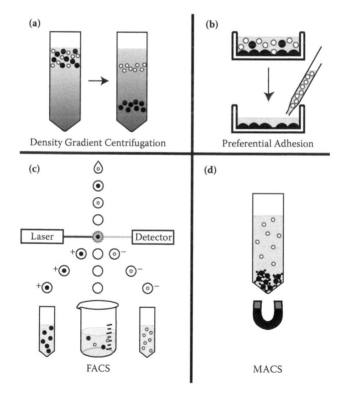

Figure 6.1
Common methods for cell separation. (a) Centrifugation separates cells based on size and density. (b) Preferential adhesion separates cells based on their intrinsic adhesive properties. (c) FACS separates cells that are bound, via specific cell surface markers, to a fluorescent tag. (d) MACS separates cells that are bound, via specific cell surface markers, to a magnetic tag.

cell population is incubated with antibodies that bind to a cell surface marker expressed only by the cells to be separated. These antibodies are conjugated to either a fluorescent probe or a magnetic bead, thus labeling the antibody-bound cells either fluorescently or magnetically.

These *tagged* cells are then separated from untagged cells via fluorescently activated cell sorting (FACS) or magnetic cell sorting (MACS) (Figure 6.1c and 6.1d, respectively). FACS is performed using a sophisticated instrument that is capable of producing a flow of tiny droplets, most containing individual cells. These droplets are excited by a laser and, based on whether the cell is tagged with fluorescently labeled antibodies or not, the droplet is electrically charged and deflected into a collection vial or waste container. In MACS, cells tagged with antibodies coupled to small magnetic beads can be pulled out of a mixed population by placing the cell suspension in a magnetic field. Cells without magnetic labels are collected in the supernatant, the magnetic field is turned off, and labeled cells are recovered.

Sorting based on cell surface markers can be performed as either *positive* isolation or *negative* isolation. In positive isolation, the target cells express the cell surface markers that are tagged by the antibody (Figure 6.2a). In negative isolation, the contaminating cells are tagged. When possible, negative isolation should be used because it requires less manipulation of the target cells (Figure 6.2b).

Yield and purity are two common measures of the effectiveness of a cell separation process. Purity is the percentage of all the cells recovered after separation that are target cells:

$$\text{Purity} = \frac{\text{target cells}_{\text{out}}}{\text{target cells}_{\text{out}} + \text{contaminating cells}_{\text{out}}} \times 100\% = \frac{\text{target cells}_{\text{out}}}{\text{total cells}_{\text{out}}} \times 100\% \quad (6.2)$$

Yield is the percentage of all the target cells present in the original, heterogeneous population that are recovered after separation:

$$\text{Yield} = \frac{\text{target cells}_{\text{out}}}{\text{target cells}_{\text{in}}} \times 100\% \quad (6.3)$$

Factors to consider when selecting the best separation method for a particular application include purity, yield, speed, cost, and required equipment.

6.2 Learning Objectives

The objectives of this experiment are to

- Practice essential lab skills including sterile technique, trypsinization, and fluorescence microscopy
- Demonstrate the principles of magnetic cell sorting to purify target cells from a heterogeneous cell population
- Quantify the effectiveness of cell separation using purity and yield

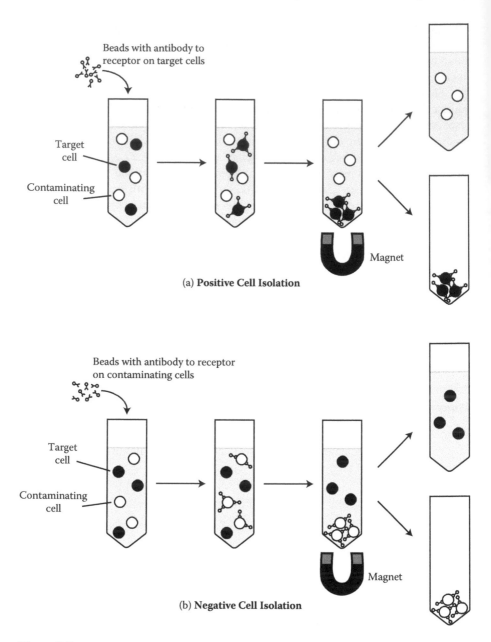

Figure 6.2
Comparison of MACS via positive and negative isolation. (a) In positive isolation, magnetic beads are conjugated to an antibody that recognizes a marker on the *target* cells. The target cells are pulled out of suspension in a magnetic field and the contaminating cells remain in the supernatant. An additional step is often needed to remove the magnetic beads from the target cells before the cells can be used. (b) In negative isolation, magnetic beads are conjugated to an antibody that recognizes a marker on the *contaminating* cells. The target cells remain in the supernatant and are untouched during the sorting process.

6.3 Overview of Experiment

Cell separation methods are typically employed to purify one cell type from a naturally heterogeneous cell population. This experiment will demonstrate the principle of magnetic sorting by intentionally creating a heterogeneous cell population by mixing cells labeled with a red or green fluorescent dye. The green cells represent the target population. The red cells represent the contaminating cell population. Contaminating cells will be captured by binding magnetic beads to their surfaces.

In practice, magnetic beads are conjugated to an antibody that binds to cell surface receptors expressed by either the contaminating cells or the target cells. In this experiment, the magnetic beads are conjugated to streptavidin, rather than an antibody. Streptavidin binds with high affinity to the small molecule biotin. Biotin can be easily attached to most proteins and will be attached to the proteins on the surface of the contaminating cells. The interaction between streptavidin and biotinylated cell surface proteins will be used to pull contaminating cells out of the heterogeneous cell suspension.

The experiment begins by labeling one flask of cells with the red fluorescent dye CMRA and a second flask with the green fluorescent dye CMFDA (Figure 6.3). If time is limited, the instructor may label the cells in advance. Next, the proteins on the surface of the red cells are covalently bound to biotin using a commercially available reagent, EZ-Link® Sulfo-NHS-LC-Biotin. The two populations of cells are combined and incubated with streptavidin-conjugated magnetic beads. The streptavidin on the beads binds, with high affinity, to the biotin on the red cells. A magnet is then used to pull these cells from the mixed population, leaving the target cells in suspension.

6.4 Safety Notes

This experiment uses a very strong magnet. Pacemakers or other implants could be damaged by exposure to the magnet. Keep magnetizable objects and delicate instruments away from the magnet. Use good lab practices and review all relevant MSDSs.

6.5 Materials

In addition to the general equipment and supplies, the following are needed to complete this experiment:

6.5.1 Reagents and Consumables

- Two flasks (T12.5 or T25) of nearly confluent 3T3 cells
- DMEM (serum free)

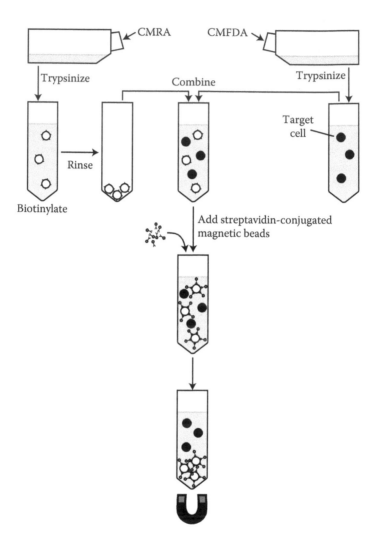

Figure 6.3
Overview of the cell separation protocol used in this experiment. Flasks of cells are labeled with either the red fluorescent dye CMRA (contaminating cells) or the green fluorescent dye CMFDA (target cells). Cell surface proteins on the contaminating cells are biotinylated before the two populations are combined. Streptavidin-conjugated magnetic beads are added to the mixed population and bind to the biotinylated, contaminating cells. A magnet pulls these cells out of suspension, leaving a purified population of target cells in the supernatant.

- 0.25% Trypsin with EDTA (1X)
- 3T3 Media (recipe follows)
- 1X Phosphate-buffered saline (PBS, pH 7.4 *and* 8.0)
- 10 mM CellTracker™ green (CMFDA, EX: 492 nm, EM: 517 nm; Molecular Probes)
- 10 mM CellTracker orange (CMRA, EX: 548 nm, EM: 576 nm; Molecular Probes)
- 0.25% Trypsin with EDTA (1X)
- EZ-Link Sulfo-NHS-LC-Biotin (Pierce Biotechnology)
- Dynabeads® M-280 streptavidin (Molecular Probes)

6.5.2 Equipment and Supplies

- DynaMag™ 15 (Molecular Probes)
- Platform rocker (temporarily housed in a refrigerator)
- Microscope equipped for fluorescence and digital imaging: a dual emission filter for concurrently viewing CMFDA (EX: 492 nm, EM: 517 nm) and CMRA (EX: 548 nm, EM: 576 nm) is suggested.

6.6 Recipes

3T3 Media. Add 50 mL bovine calf serum (BCS) and 5 mL of 100X penicillin/streptomy-cin (P/S) to 445 mL of DMEM (high glucose).

1X PBS (pH 7.4 and 8.0). Add 50 mL 10X PBS (with Ca^{2+} and Mg^{2+}) to 400 mL deion-ized H_2O (dH_2O). Mix well, adjust pH to *7.4 or 8.0* with HCl and NaOH, bring total volume to 500 mL with dH_2O, and either sterile-filter through a 0.2 µm filter or autoclave.

CMFDA. Dilute CMFDA, as supplied, to 10 mM in sterile DMSO. Store 2 µL aliquots at –20°C.

CMRA. Dilute CMRA, as supplied, to 10 mM in sterile DMSO. Store 2 µL aliquots at –20°C.

EZ-Link Sulfo-NHS-LC-Biotin. Immediately prior to use, dilute to 1 mg/mL in ice-cold PBS (pH 8.0).

6.7 Methods

6.7.1 Session 1: Sort Cells

1. In a 37°C water bath, warm ~15 mL of 3T3 media, ~5 mL of DMEM (serum free), and enough trypsin to release the plates/flasks of cells. Cool ≥40 mL of sterile PBS (pH 8.0) on ice. *Note: It is not necessary to cool the pH 7.4 PBS.*

2. Prepare the biosafety cabinet (BSC) for use by wiping it down with 70% ethanol and arranging necessary reagents and disposables. *Note: Use of the BSC is suggested to practice sterile technique and to maintain the sterility of stock solutions (as needed).*

It is not necessary to really keep the cells sterile because they will be immediately disposed of.

3. Label one plate/flask of 3T3 cells with CMRA (red fluorescent dye):

   a. Dilute 2 μL of the stock 10 mM CMRA with 2 mL of DMEM (serum free) for a final concentration of 10 μM.

   b. Aspirate media from the flask and replace with the CMRA solution.

   c. Incubate for 15–30 min at 37°C. Continue to the next step while the cells incubate with the dye.

4. Label the second plate/flask of 3T3 cells with CMFDA (green fluorescent dye):

   a. Dilute 2 μL of the stock 10 mM CMFDA with 2 mL of DMEM (serum free) for a final concentration of 10 μM.

   b. Aspirate media from the flask and replace with the CMFDA solution.

   c. Incubate for 15–30 min at 37°C. Continue to the next step while the cells incubate with the dye.

5. Biotinylate cell surface proteins on the CMRA-stained ("red") cells:

   a. Set up the microscope for fluorescence imaging; use a filter cube compatible with CMRA (EX: 548 nm, EM: 576 nm). Allow the lamp to warm up ~15 min.

   b. Remove the "red" cells from the incubator.

   c. View the cells under the microscope and verify that they fluoresce red.

   d. Remove the CMRA solution.

   e. Trypsinize the "red" cells (refer to trypsinization protocol in Appendix 1); rinse once in 10 mL 3T3 media to inactivate the trypsin and twice in 10 mL of ice-cold PBS (pH 8.0).

   f. Resuspend the cell pellet in 250 μL of 1 mg/mL EZ-Link Sulfo-NHS-LC-Biotin in ice-cold PBS (pH 8.0).

   g. Incubate for 30 min at room temperature. While waiting, trypsinize the CMFDA-treated ("green") cells as described in step 6.

6. Trypsinize the CMFDA-treated ("green") cells:

   a. Remove the "green" cells from the incubator.

   b. View the cells under the microscope and verify that they fluoresce green. Use a filter cube compatible with CMFDA (EX: 492 nm, EM: 517 nm).

   c. Remove the CMFDA solution.

   d. Trypsinize the "green" cells, rinse once in media, and spin down.

   e. Resuspend the "green" cells in 2 mL of 3T3 media.

   f. Store the "green" cell suspension in the incubator while completing Step 7.

7. After the biotinylation of the "red" cells is complete, wash them three times with 10 mL PBS (pH 7.4). After the final rinse, aspirate the supernatant but leave the pellet intact and hydrated.

8. Transfer the "green" cell suspension to the tube containing the "red" cell pellet and mix well.

9. Collect a 50 μL sample of the mixed cell suspension in a microfuge tube and set aside.

10. Incubate the cells with magnetic beads:

    a.   Add 50 μL of the Dynabeads (as supplied) to the cell suspension.

    b.   Using a rubber band, secure the tubes horizontally on a rocker platform and incubate at 4°C–8°C for 30 min. *Note: During this incubation period, you should characterize the mixed cell suspension as described next.*

11. Characterize the mixed cell suspension:

    a.   Load 10 μL of the mixed cell suspension (from step 9) in each side of a hemacytometer.

    b.   Using transmitted light and a 10X or 20X objective, focus on the cells in the center region of the grid on one side of the hemacytometer.

    c.   Switch to fluorescence imaging and count and record the number of *green* cells in the entire field of view. *Note: Remember to select the correct fluorescent filter cube to visualize the cells.*

    d.   Count and record the number of *red* cells in the entire field of view.

    e.   Repeat for the second sample on the other side of the hemacytometer. Average the counts.

12. Magnetically sort the cells:

    a.   After the 30 min incubation period with the magnetic beads, place the tube containing the mixed cell suspension on a magnet and wait 5 min.

    b.   While the tube is still in the magnetic field, carefully collect the supernatant in a conical tube.

    c.   Remove the magnet, resuspend the pellet in 2 mL of media, and collect the suspension in a separate conical tube.

13. After magnetic sorting, characterize both the cells recovered in the supernatant and the cells recovered in the pellet using a hemacytometer as described in step 11.

6.8 Data Processing and Reporting

Briefly report the results of your experiment in paragraph and graphical form. Each of the key results to report in text, figure, and/or table format is described in this section. Note that the volume of cell suspension counted on the hemacytometer was not determined. Nevertheless, the volume of cells counted and the total volume of suspension were the same for all samples. Therefore, the absolute cell counts can be compared to determine percentage purity and percentage yield.

1. Include a table, similar to Table 6.1, displaying the raw data and subsequent calculations. Show the calculations for purity and yield in the text.

2. Comment on whether or not the ratio of target cells to contaminating cells in the mixed population was as expected. If not, describe possible reasons and/or sources of error.

3. Comment on the effectiveness of the sorting technique with respect to *purity*.

4. Comment on the effectiveness of the sorting technique with respect to *yield*.

5. Compare the total number of contaminating cells recovered in the pellet and supernatant to the number present in the mixed population. Report whether or not these numbers are similar. If not, describe possible reasons and/or sources of error.

TABLE 6.1
Suggested Format for Reporting the Data

	No. Target Cells	No. Contaminating Cells
Mixed population (before sorting)		
First field of view		
Second field of view		
Mean		
Supernatant (after sorting)		
First field of view		
Second field of view		
Mean		
Pellet (after sorting)		
First field of view		
Second field of view		
Mean		
Target cell purity before sorting		—
Target cell purity after sorting		—
Target cell yield		—

6.9 Prelab Questions

1.
   a. Does the preceding protocol describe a "negative" or "positive" isolation technique? Briefly explain.

   b. Identify one major advantage of negative isolation compared to positive isolation.

2. Name one cell surface marker that is routinely used to purify hematopoietic stem cells from a mixed population. Cite your source.

3. A student wishes to purify a specific population of cells (type A) from a mixed population of cells (types A and B). Using two different separation methods, the student obtains the results illustrated in Figure 6.4.

   a. What was the yield and purity of each method, with respect to separating cell type A from the mixture?

   b. Which method (1 or 2) would be most appropriate for separating healthy bone marrow cells from contaminating tumor cells? Why?

   c. On what biochemical property of the cells is method 1 based?

   d. On what physical properties of the cells is method 2 based?

4. Review the product data sheet for the CellTracker probes used in this experiment, CMFDA and CMRA (Molecular Probes 2008).

   a. Will CMFDA and CMRA fluorescently stain dead cells? Briefly explain your answer.

   b. Do CMFDA and CMRA stain the cell membrane, nucleus, or cytoplasm?

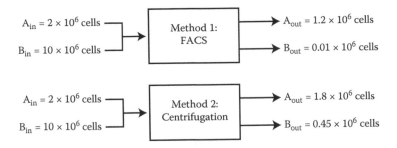

Figure 6.4
Schematic illustrating the separation of mixed cell populations using FACS and centrifugation.

    c. Why does this experiment use CellTracker dyes instead of more common fluorescent dyes—for example, calcein AM?

    d. Obtain, from your instructor, the manufacturer and catalog number for the fluorescent filter cube(s) mounted on the lab microscope, which will be used to visualize CMFDA and CMRA. For each filter cube, look up and sketch the transmission spectrum for the excitation filter, dichroic mirror, and emission filter. Identify each excitation and emission filter as a bandpass or longpass. Indicate the wavelength at which CMFDA and CMRA maximally excite and emit.

5. Residual serum-containing medium is removed from the "red" cell pellet prior to biotinylation using two consecutive rinses with 10 mL of PBS. Assume the concentration of protein in the media is 5 mg/mL and that 0.25 mL of the supernatant is retained with the pellet after each centrifugation.

    a. Calculate the residual protein, in micrograms, after two consecutive rinses with 10 mL of PBS.

    b. Calculate the residual protein, in micrograms, after one rinse with 20 mL of PBS.

    c. What volume of PBS would be needed to achieve the dilution in (a) using only one rinse?

    d. Why does the serum protein need to be removed prior to biotinylation?

6. To measure cell purity and yield, cells in the mixed population, supernatant, and pellet are loaded separately onto a hemacytometer. Standard use of a hemacytometer involves viewing the sample using transmitted light microscopy and counting the number of cells present in a specific region of the grid (refer to Appendix 2 protocol for details). In this case, the samples are viewed using fluorescence microscopy, and cells within the entire field of view are counted. Considering that the hemacytometer grid is not being used, what is the advantage of using a hemacytometer rather than, for example, adding a small volume of each sample to a multiwell plate?

6.10 Postlab Questions

1. It may be desirable to repeat the magnetic sorting step to further purify the target cell population within the supernatant. Based on your experimental results, calculate the *expected* purity and yield if the magnetic sorting is repeated (a) one more time or (b) two more times. State any assumptions made.

2. Rada, Gomes, and Reis (2011) and colleagues isolated stem cells from adipose tissue using enzymatic methods, a density gradient, or Dynabeads coated with antibodies to one of three cell surface markers (STRO-1, CD49d, or NGFr). Cell populations isolated using the different methods were compared to determine which had the greatest potential to differentiate into osteoblasts and which had the highest expression of stem cell genes.

   a. Results showed that mineralization, an indicator of osteoblast phenotype, was higher in cell populations isolated using a density gradient and enzymatic treatment than in the immunoisolated populations. What do these findings suggest about the composition of cells that would be optimum for bone tissue engineering?

   b. Additionally, the results showed that cells isolated with STRO-1 coated beads exhibited the highest expression of stem cell genes and that there were differences in gene expression among the immunoisolated populations. What do these results suggest about adipose-derived stem cells?

3. Briefly describe a tissue-engineering medical product (TEMP) on the market, in development, or completely hypothetical that incorporates magnetic cell sorting. Include the following essential components: the disease or condition the TEMP treats, the source and composition of the heterogeneous population of cells to be sorted, the cell surface marker(s) that would be used to separate the target cells, and how the purified target cells would be used in the development or manufacturing of the TEMP.

4. If you were to repeat the experiment again, what modifications would you make? Why?

References

Alberts, B., A. Johnson, J. Lewis, M. Raff, K. Roberts, and P. Walter. 2007. *Molecular biology of the cell,* 5th ed. New York: Garland Science.

Lin, K. K., and M. A. Goodell. 2011. Detection of hematopoietic stem cells by flow cytometry. In *Methods in cell biology,* eds., Darzynkiewicz, Z., E. Holden, A. Orfao, W. Telford, and D. Wlodkowic, chapter 2. New York: Academic Press.

Molecular Probes. 2008. CellTracker probes for long-term tracing of living cells. Available from http://tools.invitrogen.com/content/sfs/manuals/mp02925.pdf (accessed January 2012).

Rada, T., M. E. Gomes, and R. L. Reis. 2011. A novel method for the isolation of subpopulations of rat adipose stem cells with different proliferation and osteogenic differentiation potentials. *Journal of Tissue Engineering and Regenerative Medicine* 5 (8): 655–664.

Zuk, P. A., M. Zhu, H. Mizuno, J. Huang, J. W. Futrell, A. J. Katz, P. Benhaim, H. P. Lorenz, and M. H. Hedrick. 2001. Multilineage cells from human adipose tissue: Implications for cell-based therapies. *Tissue Engineering* 7 (2): 211–228.

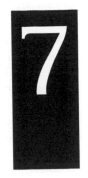

Decellularized Matrices for Tissue Engineering

7.1 Background

The extracellular matrix (ECM) provides important cues that regulate cell behavior and is unique in composition and structure for each tissue. It is difficult, if not impossible, to replicate the complexity of the native ECM when designing a scaffold for tissue engineering. A viable alternative to de novo scaffold fabrication is the removal of the primary inflammatory components (i.e., the cells) from xenogeneic and allogeneic tissues while leaving the complex ECM intact. Decellularized tissue is perhaps the best substitute for native ECM and its use has been the focus of recent clinical and research applications in tissue engineering and regenerative medicine.

Numerous decellularized ECM medical products are currently on the market, including human dermis for abdominal wall and breast reconstruction and porcine small intestinal submucosa (SIS) for general soft tissue repair and reinforcement (Keane et al. 2012). While most products on the market utilize intact decellularized tissues, it is possible to produce an injectable form of decellularized ECM that gels within the patient. The use of these injectable ECM gels as bioactive scaffold for tissue engineering is currently under investigation for treatment of myocardial infarction, traumatic injury, and urinary incontinence (Young et al. 2011; Singelyn et al. 2012; Freytes et al. 2008).

Also under development is the use of decellularized whole organs as an alternative to transplantation. Following decellularization, a donor organ would be reseeded with cells that do not cause an immune response, cultured in a bioreactor, and implanted into the patient (Song and Ott 2011; Ott et al. 2008). Decellularized tissue is also a powerful research tool. Specifically, cell culture coatings made of decellularized tissue have been explored for a variety of tissues including skin, skeletal muscle, liver, heart, and brain (DeQuach et al. 2010, 2011; Zhang et al. 2009). Compared to tissue culture plastic, these surfaces mimic the native ECM and better support adhesion, proliferation, and maintenance of cell phenotype (Zhang et al. 2009).

Methods for decellularizing tissues and organs can be characterized as physical, enzymatic, chemical, or a combination of these. *Physical* methods of decellularization include mechanical agitation, which is frequently used in conjunction with enzymatic and chemical methods, and rapid freezing to induce cell lysis (Gilbert, Sellaro, and Badylak 2006). The most common *enzymatic* decellularization protocols involve trypsin, a naturally occurring enzyme that cleaves side chains of the amino acids lysine and arginine. The enzymatic activity of trypsin is not specific for a particular protein; therefore, decellularization with trypsin can lead to a loss of laminin, fibronectin, elastin, and glycoasminoglycans (Gilbert et al. 2006). The most extensively used *chemical* method of decellularization is incubation with detergents—in particular, Triton-X and sodium dodecyl sulfate (SDS). Triton-X is a non-ionic detergent that disrupts lipid–lipid and lipid–protein interactions but should not affect protein–protein interactions. SDS is an ionic detergent that does affect protein–protein interactions and, as a result, may disrupt native structure more than Triton-X (Gilbert et al. 2006). Many variables influence the efficacy of any decellularization protocol, including method, treatment time, and the size, composition, and structure of the tissue to be decellularized.

The efficacy of a decellularization protocol depends on both the removal of cellular contents and the retention of tissue-specific ECM. To assess removal of cellular contents, histology and fluorescent DNA-binding dyes can be used to visualize any remaining nuclei within the decellularized tissue. To visualize cell nuclei using histology, decellularized tissue sections can be cut on a microtome or cryostat, stained with hematoxylin and eosin (H&E), and viewed using transmitted light microscopy. H&E is a classic histology method that stains nuclei blue/purple against a background of proteins stained pink/orange. As an alternative to H&E, tissue sections can be stained with a DNA-binding fluorescent dye, such as Hoechst 33258 (EX: 352 nm, EM: 461 nm) and viewed using fluorescent microscopy. To quantify the DNA remaining in a decellularized tissue, a sample can be enzymatically digested and then a DNA assay, such a PicoGreen®, can be performed to measure the DNA concentration in the digest.

Histology, immunohistochemistry, gel electrophoresis, mass spectroscopy, and biochemical assays can be used to characterize the composition and organization of the ECM that remains following decellularization. Mechanical testing of the decellularized tissue is also important when the tissue plays a structural role in the body.

7.2 Learning Objectives

The objectives of this experiment are to

- Compare the effectiveness of two protocols for decellularizing porcine skeletal muscle tissue
- Gain experience using histology to characterize engineered and native tissues

7.3 Overview of Experiment

This experiment compares the effectiveness of two protocols for decellularizing tissue. The two protocols are identical except that the detergent used is either Triton-X

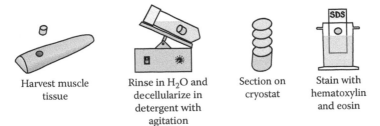

Harvest muscle tissue · Rinse in H₂O and decellularize in detergent with agitation · Section on cryostat · Stain with hematoxylin and eosin

Figure 7.1
Schematic of the decellularization experiment that will be performed in this lab. Porcine skeletal muscle is cored, rinsed, and decellularized by incubating it in detergent for 48 h with agitation. Finally, decellularized samples and untreated samples are sectioned on a cryostat and stained with H&E to compare the effectiveness of the decellularization protocols.

or SDS. Porcine skeletal muscle will be cored (Figure 7.1a), rinsed, and then decellularized by incubating it in detergent for 48 h with agitation (Figure 7.1b). In sessions 2 and 3, the samples will be frozen and sectioned on a cryostat in preparation for histological evaluation (Figure 7.1c). In the final session, the samples will be stained with H&E to visually determine the effectiveness of the decellularization protocols (Figure 7.1d).

7.4 Safety Notes

This protocol utilizes chemicals that are classified as serious fire hazards. Carefully review all relevant MSDSs and use proper personal protective equipment. The cryostat blade is extremely sharp, so use caution when setting up the equipment and sectioning samples.

7.5 Materials

In addition to the general equipment and supplies, the following are needed to complete the experiment:

7.5.1 Reagents and Consumables

- Porcine skeletal muscle (pork tenderloin; ~15 cm² × 2 cm) *Note: Avoid water- and/or brine-injected pork if possible. The tenderloin should be cut lengthwise, as needed, to achieve approximate desired thickness.*
- 1.2 cm diameter sterile biopsy punch
- Phosphate-buffered saline (PBS) + 1% penicillin/streptomycin (P/S)
- Triton X-100

- Sodium dodecyl sulfate (SDS)
- Optional: ethidium homodimer (EthD-1)
- Tissue Tek O.C.T.
- Disposable cryomolds
- Dry ice
- Microscope slides with frosted ends
- Hematoxylin solution (gill formulation #1, 2 g/L)
- Bluing reagent (e.g., Fisher Scientific protocol bluing reagent)
- Eosin Y (0.5% solution)
- 70% Ethanol (EtOH)
- 90% EtOH
- 100% EtOH
- Histo-Clear
- Histomount
- Glass coverslips

7.5.2 Equipment and Supplies

- Platform rocker
- Cryogloves
- Styrofoam cooler
- Cryostat
- Slide storage box
- Chemical fume hood
- Tissue-Tek slide staining station
- 24-Slide holder with handle
- Microscope equipped for color digital imaging (optional activity requires fluorescent imaging capabilities; EX: 528 nm, EM: 617 nm)

7.6 Recipes

1X PBS. Add 50 mL 10X PBS (with Ca^{2+} and Mg^{2+}) to 400 mL deionized water (dH_2O). Mix well, adjust pH to 7.4 with HCl and NaOH, and bring total volume to 500 mL with dH_2O.

PBS + 1% P/S. Add 1 mL of P/S for every 99 mL of PBS.

1% Triton X. Add 1 mL of Triton X-100 for every 99 mL PBS + 1% P/S. Filter-sterilize.

1% SDS. Dissolve 1 g of SDS per 100 mL of PBS + 1% P/S. Filter-sterilize.

70% and 90% EtOH. Dilute 100% EtOH with dH_2O.

7.7 Methods

7.7.1 Session 1: Prepare Samples and Begin the Decellularization Process*

1. Prepare the biosafety cabinet (BSC) for use by wiping it down with 70% ethanol and arranging necessary reagents and disposables.

2. Working on a sterile surface within the BSC, such as the inside of a petri dish, use a sterile biopsy punch to cut six full-thickness samples out of the pork tenderloin. Avoid any visibly fatty regions of the tissue.

3. Record observations about the integrity, size, and shape of the samples in your lab notebook.

4. Label two conical tubes, "untreated." Place two of the samples in the tubes and directly into the freezer.

5. Rinse the remaining samples:

   a. Place each of the remaining samples into a separate 50 mL conical tube.

   b. Add 40 mL of sterile deionized water (dH$_2$O) to each tube and cap tightly.

   c. Using a rubber band, secure the tubes horizontally on a rocker platform and agitate for 30 min. at room temperature (RT).

   d. Remove the dH$_2$O.

6. Add either 20 mL of sterile 1% Triton-X ($n = 2$) or sterile 1% SDS ($n = 2$) to each tube. Label them accordingly.

7. Place the four tubes back on the rocker and agitate at room temperature (RT) for ~48 h. Record the exact length of time in your notebook.

8. (Optional) Stain a representative piece of tissue:

   a. Examine the remnants of the tissue from which the cores were cut and try to determine the predominant muscle fiber orientation.

   b. With a scalpel, carefully cut a few thin slices of the tissue along the direction of the fibers. Make the slices as thin as possible for optimal imaging.

   c. Place the slices in a multiwell plate and add 200 μL of PBS plus 2 μL of EthD-1.

   d. Cover the plate to protect the samples from light and incubate for 10 min at RT.

   e. Using forceps, take one or more tissue slices out of the dye and position them in the center of a clean microscope slide. Transfer just enough liquid to keep the tissue hydrated while avoiding the risk of the liquid running off the slide and onto the microscope.

   f. Place the slide on the microscope stage, select the filter cube that is compatible with a red dye (EX: 528 nm, EM: 617 nm), and view the sample using fluorescence microscopy. The *nucleus* of dead cells will fluoresce red because EthD-1 crosses damaged cell membranes and activates after binding to DNA. Try to find a region

---

* This session may be performed on the lab bench; however, doing so may result in significant bacterial growth during the decellularization process.

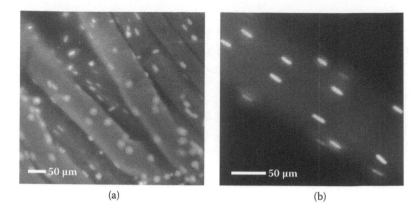

(a)   (b)

Figure 7.2
Micrograph of a piece of pork tenderloin stained with EthD-1. Images were captured using fluorescence microscopy and a 20X (a) or 40X (b) objective. The parallel arrangement of muscle fibers and elongated shape of the cell nuclei are evident.

of the sample where the parallel arrangement of muscle fibers is evident and note the elongated shape of the nuclei (Figure 7.2).

7.7.2 Session 2: Embed Samples for Sectioning on the Cryostat

1. Remove the two untreated samples from the freezer and bring to RT.
2. Remove the decellularized samples from the rocker and aspirate off the solution containing the cellular remnants.
3. Rinse the decellularized samples with 40 mL dH$_2$O three times, shaking the tube vigorously with each rinse.
4. Carefully blot the samples on a lint-free wiper.
5. In your lab notebook, record any observations about the integrity, size, and shape of the different samples. Note any regional variability that exists within a sample. If possible, take a photo of the samples to document your observations further.
6. Embed the samples for sectioning:
   a. Arrange six plastic cryomolds on the lab bench.
   b. Using a lab marker, label each mold "untreated," "SDS," or "Triton-X."
   c. Place a small drop of Tissue Tek O.C.T. in the center of each mold.
   d. Using forceps, place the samples in the center of the appropriate mold. Gently spread the samples out flat in the center of the mold, being careful not to tear the tissue.
   e. Fill the mold, until it is just level, with Tissue Tek O.C.T. Be careful not to create bubbles during this process.

7. Using the cryogloves, place the block of dry ice in the base of a Styrofoam cooler. Carefully set the molds on top of the dry ice block and wait until the embedding medium freezes completely. Alternatively, place the samples in the −80°C freezer until they are completely frozen.

8. Section the samples as described next or store them frozen until needed.

7.7.3 Session 3: Cryosection Samples

The following is a set of general instructions for using a cryostat. For additional details, refer to the manufacturer's instructions for the specific cryostat you are using.

1. Set the temperature of the cryostat to −20°C and wait for the sectioning chamber to reach −20°C.

2. If the samples are being stored at −80°C, place them in the cryostat to bring them to −20°C. Initially, only one sample per group (untreated, Triton X, and SDS) is needed. The duplicate samples will be used in the event that there is a problem with the first sample.

3. While the chamber and samples are coming to temperature, label the frosted portion of the slides with a *pencil*. Label four slides each for untreated, Triton X, and SDS.

4. Attach the untreated sample to the chuck:

   a. Remove one of the untreated samples from its mold by inverting onto a surface.

   b. Spread a thin layer of O.C.T. on the chuck.

   c. Keeping the sample in the same orientation (surface that was at the bottom of the mold is now facing up), gently press the sample into the O.C.T.

   d. Add a little more O.C.T. around the perimeter of the sample.

   e. Allow the O.C.T. to freeze, securing the sample onto the chuck.

5. Cover the bottom surface of the cryostat with plastic wrap. This will make cleanup much easier.

6. Secure the chuck onto the stage and retract the stage fully.

7. Very carefully, secure the blade in the blade holder.

8. Bring the sample forward, close to the blade, and align the sample parallel with the blade.

9. Set the thickness of the samples to 10 μm.

10. Cut a few sections and adjust the stage, as needed, so that the blade travels evenly across the entire face of the sample.

11. Continue cutting sections until a significant portion of the tissue is visible. At that point, brush off any debris from the blade or sample.

12. Position the roll bar on top of the cutting platform and cut a section. Lift the roll bar. If the sample looks good, bring the top surface of a glass slide (the labeled side) close to the section. The slide will lift the section off the platform and onto the slide.

13. Continue sectioning until you make four high-quality slides of the untreated tissue.

14. Repeat steps 4–13 for the Triton X and SDS samples. Use the spare samples in the freezer as needed.

15. Place the slides and extra samples in a slide storage box in the freezer at −20° or −80°C until session 4.

16. Clean up the cryostat:

    a. Carefully remove the blade. If the blade is disposable, throw it away in a sharps container. If not, carefully wipe it with ethanol and return it to its storage box.

    b. Throw the plastic wrap with all the extra shavings away.

    c. Wipe all the surfaces with ethanol.

7.7.4 Session 4: Perform Histology

1. Cover the work surface of a fume hood with absorbent bench paper. Place the slide staining station on the paper and fill the staining dishes from left (dish 1) to right (dish 9) as indicated in Table 7.1. *Note: The staining station may be set up in advance by the instructors.*

2. Place a large beaker (~1 L) filled with dH_2O and the bottle of Histomount in the fume hood.

3. Load the slides into the slide holder.

4. Submerge the slide holder and slides in each solution as specified, starting with dish 1 and continuing in the order indicated (Table 7.1).

5. After staining is complete, mount the slides:

    a. Lay the slides out on a level surface in the fume hood.

    b. Place one drop of Histomount near the edge of each piece of tissue.

    c. Place a glass coverslip on top of each slide, covering the tissue and spreading out the Histomount (Figure 7.3).

TABLE 7.1
Protocol for Staining with H&E[a]

Container	Reagent	Staining Time or Number of Dips
Dish 1	dH_2O	3 min
Dish 2	Hematoxylin[b]	5 min
Dish 3	dH_2O	1 dip
Large beaker	dH_2O	3 min
Dish 4	Bluing reagent[b]	15 dips
Dish 5	Eosin[b]	1 min
Dish 6	70% EtOH	2 dips
Dish 7	90% EtOH	3 dips
Dish 8	100% EtOH	1 min
Dish 9	Histo-Clear	1.5 min

[a] Submerge the slides in each solution starting with dish 1 and continuing in the order indicated for the duration indicated.
[b] Reagents are toxic and should be capped when not in use.

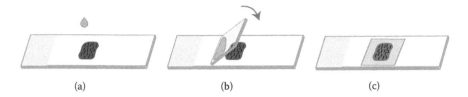

Figure 7.3
Schematic illustrating a technique for mounting the coverslip on the slide without creating air bubbles in the sample.

    d.   Carefully force out any bubbles using a pipette tip.

    e.   Allow to dry for 30 min.

6. Cap or properly dispose of the staining solutions in the slide staining station. The dH_2O *in the beaker,* which contains trace hematoxylin, can be emptied down the drain while flushing with water. The other solutions should be reused or collected as hazardous waste and disposed of according to local regulations.

7. Visualize the slides on the microscope using transmitted light. Look at various regions of each sample to ascertain the extent of decellularization. Capture *representative* images of each sample using a high- and low-powered objective.

8. Obtain a calibration image so that you will be able to add a scale bar to representative micrographs when documenting your results. You may get a calibration image from your instructor or acquire an image of a stage micrometer or hemacytometer grid using the same magnification as in the micrographs.

7.8 Data Processing and Reporting

Each of the key results to report in text, figure, and/or table format is described next.

1. Summarize any changes you observed in the size, shape, and/or integrity of the samples after decellularization. Note any differences in the samples from the two decellularization protocols or any regional variability within a single sample. If photos were taken, include them.

2. Include one high-quality figure with *representative* micrographs of untreated, Triton-X decellularized, and SDS decellularized samples stained with H&E. Include a scale bar and mark any nuclei visible in the decellularized samples with an asterisk.

3. Comment on the relative effectiveness of the decellularization methods based on the histology results.

7.9 Prelab Questions

1. The first step in the decellularization protocol is to rinse the tissue in dH_2O. What affect will dH_2O have on the cells residing in the tissue? Briefly explain.

2. Calculate the molarity of the 1% SDS solution (MW = 288.38).

3. Briefly describe the primary function/mode of action of each of the following reagents in the staining protocol: hematoxylin, bluing reagent, eosin, EtOH rinses, and Histo-Clear. Cite your sources.

4. The numerical aperture (NA) quantifies the ability of a microscope objective to collect the light coming from the specimen and is given by the following expression:

$$NA = n \sin \alpha \qquad (7.1)$$

where n is the refractive index through which the light is traveling and α is half of the angle formed by the cone of light between the objective and sample. The refractive indexes of air and oil are 1.0 and 1.5, respectively. The smallest distance (r) between objects that can be fully resolved is estimated by

$$r = \frac{0.5\lambda}{NA} = \frac{0.5\lambda}{n \sin \alpha} \qquad (7.2)$$

where λ is the wavelength of light forming the image. Visible, white light is centered at a wavelength of 550 nm.

a. Is a high or low NA desirable in a microscope objective? Briefly explain.

b. Imagine that, in the course of this experiment, you are analyzing a tissue sample that has two nuclei in near proximity. Assume the nuclei are perfectly round with a diameter of 1 μm. How far apart do the centers of the nuclei need to be to resolve them if your objective has an NA of 0.40?

7.10 Postlab Questions

1. Read the paper by DeQuach and colleagues (2010) entitled "Simple and High Yielding Method for Preparing Specific Extracellular Matrix Coating for Cell Culture."

    a. Based on their findings, what *structural proteins* would you expect to be present in the ECM of your samples after decellularization with SDS?

    b. Identify a technique that would allow you to confirm the presence of these proteins visually in your sectioned tissue.

2. A review of methods for decellularizing tissues states that results with Triton-X have been "mixed" (Gilbert, Sellaro, and Badylak 2006). What features of the tissue and what experimental variables may contribute to the effectiveness, or lack of effectiveness, of Triton-X?

3. What might be the consequence of not fully removing cellular remnants during manufacturing of a TEMP?

4. Estimate the density of nuclei in the porcine skeletal muscle tissue (per cubic centimeter tissue) from the micrographs of the untreated samples. State any assumptions you make.

References

DeQuach, J. A., V. Mezzano, A. Miglani, S. Lange, G. M. Keller, F. Sheikh, and K. L. Christman. 2010. Simple and high yielding method for preparing tissue specific extracellular matrix coatings for cell culture. *PloS One* 5 (9): e13039.

DeQuach, J. A., S. H. Yuan, L. S. Goldstein, and K. L. Christman. 2011. Decellularized porcine brain matrix for cell culture and tissue engineering scaffolds. *Tissue Engineering. Part A* 17 (21–22): 2583–2592.

Freytes, D. O., J. Martin, S. S. Velankar, A. S. Lee, and S. F. Badylak. 2008. Preparation and rheological characterization of a gel form of the porcine urinary bladder matrix. *Biomaterials* 29 (11): 1630–1637.

Gilbert, T. W., T. L. Sellaro, and S. F. Badylak. 2006. Decellularization of tissues and organs. *Biomaterials* 27 (19): 3675–3683.

Keane, T. J., R. Londono, N. J. Turner, and S. F. Badylak. 2012. Consequences of ineffective decellularization of biologic scaffolds on the host response. *Biomaterials* 33 (6): 1771–1781.

Ott, H. C., T. S. Matthiesen, S. K. Goh, L. D. Black, S. M. Kren, T. I. Netoff, and D. A. Taylor. 2008. Perfusion-decellularized matrix: using nature's platform to engineer a bioartificial heart. *Nature Medicine* 14 (2): 213–221.

Singelyn, J. M., P. Sundaramurthy, T. D. Johnson, P. J. Schup-Magoffin, D. P. Hu, D. M. Faulk, J. Wang, et al. 2012. Catheter-deliverable hydrogel derived from decellularized ventricular extracellular matrix increases endogenous cardiomyocytes and preserves cardiac function post-myocardial infarction. *Journal of the American College of Cardiology* 59:751–763.

Song, J. J., and H. C. Ott. 2011. Organ engineering based on decellularized matrix scaffolds. *Trends in Molecular Medicine* 17 (8): 424–432.

Young, D. A., D. O. Ibrahim, D. Hu, and K. L. Christman. 2011. Injectable hydrogel scaffold from decellularized human lipoaspirate. *Acta Biomaterica* 7 (3): 1040–1049.

Zhang, Y., Y. He, S. Bharadwaj, N. Hammam, K. Carnagey, R. Myers, A. Atala, and M. Van Dyke. 2009. Tissue-specific extracellular matrix coatings for the promotion of cell proliferation and maintenance of cell phenotype. *Biomaterials* 30 (23–24): 4021–4028.

Chapter 8

Effect of Plating Density on Cell Adhesion to Varied Culture Matrices

8.1 Background

Cell adhesion is a complex event that refers to binding of cells to a surface. This surface may be another cell, the surrounding extracellular matrix (ECM), or an artificial scaffold. Mammalian cells coexist *in vivo* in intimate contact with each other and the surrounding ECM, and adhesion between these surfaces is directed at the molecular level by two different types of interactions. "Cell–cell adhesion" is regulated by membrane expression of specialized integral membrane proteins called *cell adhesion molecules* (CAMs) that are generally clustered together at specialized points of cell contact. Cell–cell adhesion links the cytoplasm of neighboring cells and can regulate signal transduction (Clark and Brugge 1995; Pardi 2010; Aplin, Howe, and Juliano 1999). However, cells also adhere indirectly by binding of membrane *adhesion receptors* to specified components of the ECM ("cell–matrix adhesion").

By way of these two types of interactions, cells can communicate bidirectionally with each other and respond to changes in the extracellular environment (Miranti and Brugge 2002). The process of adhesion regulates cell shape and biomechanics and is required for a variety of other cellular processes, including proliferation, differentiation, migration, invasion, embryogenesis, wound healing, and tissue remodeling as well as maintenance of three-dimensional multicellular tissues and organs (Kim 2011). Therefore, control of cellular adhesion has important technological applications in the design and use of devices for stem cell isolation or scaffolds used in tissue repair.

The ECM is an organized network of proteins and polysaccharides secreted by cells that play a key regulatory role in determining the development, organization, and biological behavior of cells. In mammalian systems, three types of molecules are abundant in the ECM of all tissues: collagens, multiadhesive matrix proteins, and proteoglycans (Figure 8.1). While collagen fibers and proteoglycans provide mechanical support, it is primarily the adhesive matrix proteins that bind to cell-surface adhesion receptors and other ECM components.

Cultured cells exhibit variable responses to different ECM components depending upon membrane expression levels of these adhesion receptors, as demonstrated by a study that examined the behavior of mouse embryonic stem (ES) cells seeded within scaffolds containing the matrix components fibronectin and laminin (Battista et al. 2005). Fibronectin promoted differentiation of ES cells into endothelial cells, while addition of laminin promoted differentiation of the same ES cells into cardiomyocytes. Matrix components can therefore be a useful tool to direct cellular behaviors in tissue and regenerative engineering studies. *In vitro* modulation of ECMs has several functions, including provision of a defined cell-adhesive substrate, control over three-dimensional tissue structure, and presentation of relevant signals (including growth factors, cell-adhesion molecules, and mechanical signals) (Kim 2011).

The design criteria for artificial ECMs can vary considerably depending on the desired engineered tissue. Researchers must therefore be cognizant as to how cells differentially react to their microenvironment and advantageously use this to regulate cellular adhesion. A suboptimal substrate may result in inefficient adhesion, poor cellular response, or inclusion of inappropriate cell numbers and reagents in order to achieve the desired outcome. Consequently, it is desirable to optimize cell adhesion in scaffold- or transplant-based experiments.

This lab examines differential adhesion responses to two protein-based, natural biomaterials that are abundant *in vivo* and form the basic network of the cellular basement membrane (basal lamina): collagen type IV and laminin (Figure 8.1). The basal lamina is a network of ECM components that supports epithelial sheets and surrounds most groups of cells (i.e., four to eight cell embryos, fat, muscle, etc.), thereby playing an important role in embryonic development and tissue repair. Collagens are the most abundant component of connective tissue, and collagen type IV forms the base of the basement membrane to influence cell adhesion and survival

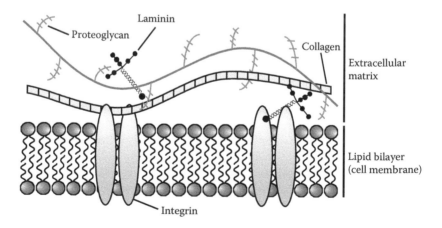

Figure 8.1
Extracellular adhesive protein interaction with the cell membrane.

(Kruegel and Miosge 2010). Laminins are a class of multifunctional glycoproteins that provides a protein network in the basal lamina. Laminins are often used to culture and maintain differentiated cellular phenotype, but are also shown to influence adhesion and cell migration (Gu et al. 2003).

Because these natural biomaterials are found *in vivo*, they are attractive in terms of tissue regeneration strategies (stem cell differentiation and transplantation) because they exhibit appropriately defined biological properties (including cell adhesion), exhibit mechanical properties similar to those of natural tissues, are biodegradable, and exhibit excellent biocompatibility (Kim 2011). Nevertheless, it is important to remember that often synthetic polymers are used *in vitro* to create more specifically controlled cellular responses because they may be purer and therefore less likely to induce inflammatory responses, particularly in transplantation studies.

8.2 Learning Objectives

The objectives of this experiment are to

- Investigate the effectiveness of individual matrix components in supporting L929 cellular adhesion
- Examine the impact of cellular plating density on different substrates
- Consider improvements to the design of this type of experimental protocol

8.3 Overview of Experiment

The overall procedure for this experiment involves precoating the wells of a non-treated 96-well assay plate with different ECM substrates. Cells are plated at various densities (0.25×10^6, 0.1×10^6, and 0.25×10^5 cells/well) and allowed a defined period of time to adhere. The number of adherent cells is determined postfixation using a colorimetric assay in order to determine substrate differences in promoting adhesion of L929 fibroblasts (Figure 8.2).

8.4 Safety Notes

Use good lab practices and review all relevant MSDSs. When preparing collagen, dilute acetic acid in the fume hood and wear appropriate personal protective equipment including goggles, gloves, and lab coat.

8.5 Materials

In addition to the general equipment and supplies, the following are needed to complete this experiment:

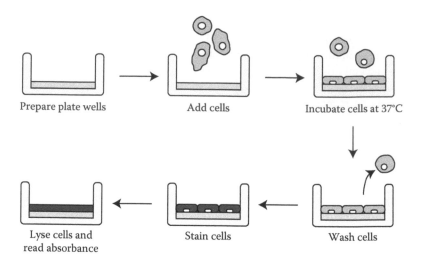

Figure 8.2
Overview of the experimental protocol.

8.5.1 Reagents and Consumables

- 1% Bovine serum albumin (BSA)
- 96-Well assay plate (flat-bottom, low evaporation lid, nontreated, sterile)
- 0.1% Poly-l-lysine
- 1X Phosphate-buffered saline (PBS)
- 100 µg/mL Laminin (from basement membrane)
- 1 mg/mL Collagen type IV in 0.25% acetic acid
- 2% Paraformaldehyde
- >10 × 10^6 L929 Fibroblasts in monolayer culture (e.g., 3 × 100 mm confluent dishes)
- L929 Media (recipe follows)
- 0.25% Trypsin with EDTA (1X)
- Trypan blue
- Toluidine blue
- 1% Triton-X

8.5.2 Equipment and Supplies

- 12-Channel pipettor (30–300 µL)
- Belly Dancer™ orbital shaker
- Microplate reader (to measure absorbance at 590 nm) with acquisition software

8.6 Recipes

1X PBS. Add 50 mL 10X PBS (with Ca^{2+} and Mg^{2+}) to 400 mL deionized H_2O (dH_2O). Mix well, adjust pH to 7.4 with HCl and NaOH, bring total volume to 500 mL with dH_2O, and either sterile-filter through a 0.2 µm filter or autoclave.

1% BSA. Dissolve 0.1 g of BSA in 10 mL of PBS. Gently mix by rocking at 4°C. Once dissolved, sterile-filter using a 0.2 µm syringe filter and store at 4°C. Do not use stored solution if residual, nondissolved BSA is visible by eye.

L929 Media. Add 50 mL bovine calf serum (BCS) and 5 mL of 100X penicillin/streptomycin (P/S) to 445 mL of high glucose DMEM.

50 mM Tris/HCl-150 mM NaCl (pH 7.5; for diluting laminin). Add 0.61 g of Tris base and 0.88 g of NaCl to 80 mL of dH_2O. Mix well and adjust the pH to 7.5 using HCl. Bring the final volume to 100 mL using dH_2O.

Laminin (per manufacturer's instructions). Thaw laminin slowly on ice. Dilute to working concentration (100 µg/mL) in sterile-filtered 50 mM Tris/HCl-150 mM NaCl (pH 7.5). Prepare 650 µL aliquots in microfuge tubes prechilled on ice and store at –20°C. Thaw laminin aliquots on ice prior to experimental use.

Collagen type IV (per manufacturer's instructions). Thaw stock collagen type IV on ice. Resuspend to 1 mg/mL in 0.25% acetic acid (handle carefully in the fume hood and wear appropriate personal protective equipment). Aliquot to microfuge tubes prechilled on ice and store at 4°C. Keep aliquot on ice during experimental use.

Toluidine blue. Prepare as 0.2% solution in PBS. Mix well by shaking at room temperature (RT) on an orbital shaker. Sterile-filter using a 0.2 µm syringe filter and store at RT.

2% Paraformaldehyde. Measure 2 g of paraformaldehyde and add to 100 mL of PBS. Heat to 55°C–60°C to dissolve and add several drops of 1 N NaOH until the solution becomes clear. Remove from heat and allow solution to cool before adjusting the pH to 7.2–7.4. Prepare small-volume aliquots, wrap in aluminum foil, and store at –20°C. Thawed aliquots can be stored at 4°C for up to 1 month.

8.7 Methods

8.7.1 Session 1: Prepare Substrate-Coated Culture Assay Plate

1. Prepare the BSC for use by wiping down with 70% ethanol and arranging necessary reagents and disposables.

2. Inside the BSC, prepare 0.01% poly-l-lysine by adding 1 mL of stock 0.1% poly-l-lysine to 9 mL of sterile-filtered PBS in a sterile 15 mL conical tube and mixing thoroughly by rotating on an orbital shaker.

3. Continue to work inside the BSC and remove one 96-well assay plate from its packaging. Label the plate lid with your name, the date, and assigned substrate columns (Figure 8.3).

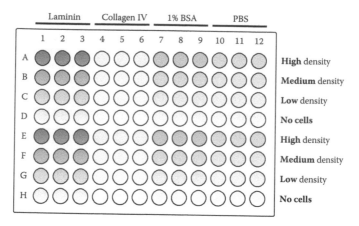

Figure 8.3
Suggested cell adhesion culture plate template.

4. Remove the assay plate lid and set aside. Use a multichannel pipettor to transfer 50 µL of poly-l-lysine solution into each well in the 96-well plate. Replace the lid of the assay plate, tap the plate gently to ensure the bottoms of the wells are covered with poly-l-lysine, and leave the plate in the hood for 30 min at RT.

5. Obtain a bucket of ice. Place one aliquot of 100 µg/mL laminin on ice to thaw slowly (obtain from your instructor).

6. After the 30 min incubation, remove the plate lid and wash all wells coated with poly-l-lysine by adding 150 µL sterile PBS per well (use the multichannel pipettor). Gently swirl the plate to ensure that the wells are adequately rinsed and invert on a stack of paper towels. Capillary action will cause the PBS wash to come out of the wells, although you may need to tap the plate *gently* against the paper towels several times to ensure removal of all wash buffer.

7. Wash the wells a second time with PBS.

8. Place the assay plate on ice and add 25 µL of laminin, collagen type IV, or 1% BSA to the appropriately labeled wells (refer to Figure 8.3). PBS should be added to the control wells to retain hydration equivalent to the other wells. Replace the lid of the assay plate and gently swirl the plate to ensure that the wells are evenly coated. Place the plate into the 37°C incubator.

9. After 1 h, remove the assay plate from the incubator. In the BSC, add 150 µL of 1X sterile PBS to each well and gently swirl. Invert the plate on a stack of paper towels to remove the PBS wash. Wash the wells two more times with PBS.

10. Replace the lid on the assay plate and seal the edges with parafilm. Place the sealed plate into a plastic sandwich bag and store at 4°C until the next laboratory session. The wells do not need to be kept hydrated at this point.

8.7.2 Session 2: Plate Cells and Determine Matrix Adhesion

1. Prepare the BSC for use by wiping down with 70% ethanol and arranging necessary reagents and disposables.

2. Place an aliquot of 2% paraformaldehyde in a 37°C water bath to prewarm. The paraformaldehyde solution may need to be vortexed to ensure that all powder has redissolved.

3. Remove the 96-well assay plate from storage and the plastic bag. Place the plate into the 37°C incubator to prewarm. While at the incubator, remove the L929 cells. If the cells are provided in suspension, skip step 4.

4. Prepare L929 cells:

   a. View the cells under the microscope. In your lab notebook, note the appearance and confluence of the cells.

   b. Trypsinize the cells (refer to trypsinization protocol in Appendix 1).

   c. Spin the cell suspension down in a centrifuge at 300 g, discard the supernatant, and resuspend the pellet in 2–3 mL of L929 media.

   d. Count the cells using a hemacytometer (refer to cell counting protocol in Appendix 2).

   e. Dilute the cell suspension to achieve a concentration of 2.5×10^6 cells/mL of media (high density of cells). You will need at least 4 mL of this suspension.

   f. In separate 15 mL conical tubes, prepare dilutions of 1.0×10^6 cells/mL (mid-density) and 2.5×10^5 cells/mL (low density). Plan the dilutions so that you have at least 2.5 mL of each suspension density (high, medium, and low). Record your calculations in your lab notebook. Set the cells aside in the BSC.

5. Remove the lid of the assay plate and rinse each well one time with 150 μL sterile PBS.

6. Pipette 100 μL of each cell dilution to the appropriate wells (refer to Figure 8.3).

7. Add 100 μL of culture media (no cells) to the control wells.

8. Return the assay plate to the 37°C incubator and allow the cells to adhere for 1 h.

9. After 1 h, remove the plate from the incubator and return to the BSC. Invert the plate on a stack of paper towels to remove excess media.

10. *Carefully* wash each well with 150 μL PBS to remove nonadherent cells. It is important that the wells not be allowed to dry out from this point forward.

11. Add 30 μL 2% prewarmed paraformaldehyde to each well and fix for 15 min at RT.

12. Wash each well three times with 150 μL PBS as previously described.

13. Stain adherent cells by adding 50 μL 0.2% toluidine blue to each well (including the control wells, which do not contain any cells). Gently rotate the plate for 30 min at RT on an orbital shaker.

14. Wash each well five times with 150 μL PBS.

15. *If time allows, view the samples using a light microscope to assess differences visually in adherent cell number between wells. Use image capture software to acquire representative images of cells adhering to different substrates. Obtain a calibration image so that you will be able to add a scale bar to representative micrographs when documenting your results. You may get a calibration image from your instructor or acquire an image of a stage micrometer or hemacytometer grid using the same magnification as in the micrographs.*

16. Add 100 μL 1% Triton-X carefully to each well. Rotate the plate on the orbital shaker for 30 min (RT) to lyse cells.

17. While the samples are lysing, turn the microplate reader on and set the absorbance wavelength to 590 nm.

18. When sample lysing is complete, insert the plate into the microplate reader and use the associated software to determine sample absorbance values. Ensure that the underside of the plate is clear of fingerprints or other residue (which may distort absorbance readings) by wiping with a lab tissue.

19. Record the absorbance values in your lab notebook.

20. Dispose of the assay plate according to appropriate waste disposal procedures and clean up your workstation.

8.8 Data Processing and Reporting

Briefly report the results of your experiment in paragraph and graphical form. Each of the key results to report in the text, figure, and/or table format is described next.

1. Show your calculations for determining total cell number and consequent cell sample dilutions.

2. Prepare a bar graph showing the trends in cell adhesion for the different concentrations of cell samples on the different matrices. Include error bars and label appropriately.

3. Statistical analysis: perform a one-way ANOVA on the preceding data to determine the effect of cell density on adherence to each matrix substrate. Report the degrees of freedom, critical F-value corresponding to $p < 0.05$, the p-value obtained from your data, and the statistical power. Use an appropriate post hoc test to examine pairwise differences.

4. *If time allowed microscopic analysis,* include representative images of adherent cells on each substrate. Be sure to include appropriate scale bars and labels.

8.9 Prelab Questions

1. Why does the protocol include a cell lysing step?
2. Why is it important to use PBS containing calcium and magnesium?
3. Why is a standard curve not included in this protocol?
4. Predict how collagen type IV and laminin differentially affect cell adhesion.
5. Name three other matrix substrates that could be examined in this assay.

8.10 Postlab Questions

1. Does this type of assay provide good reproducibility?
2. Do the cells adhere equally to each matrix? Why or why not?
3. How does plating density affect cell adhesion? Is this trend observed on all matrix substrates examined?
4. What are the advantages to being able to control cell adhesion?

References

Aplin, A. E., A. K. Howe, and R. L. Juliano. 1999. Cell adhesion molecules, signal transduction and cell growth. *Current Opinion in Cell Biology* 11 (6): 737–744.

Battista, S., D. Guarnieri, C. Borselli, S. Zeppetelli, A. Borzacchiello, L. Mayol, D. Gerbasio, D. R. Keene, L. Ambrosio, and P. A. Netti. 2005. The effect of matrix composition of 3D constructs on embryonic stem cell differentiation. *Biomaterials* 26 (31): 6194–6207.

Clark, E. A., and J. S. Brugge. 1995. Integrins and signal transduction pathways: The road taken. *Science* 268 (5208): 233–239.

Gu, Y. C., J. Kortesmaa, K. Tryggvason, J. Persson, P. Ekblom, S. E. Jacobsen, and M. Ekblom. 2003. Laminin isoform-specific promotion of adhesion and migration of human bone marrow progenitor cells. *Blood* 101 (3): 877–885.

Kim, B-S., I-K. Park, T. Hoshiba, H-L. Jiang, Y-J. Choi, T. Akaike, and C-S. Cho. 2011. Design of artificial extracellular matrices for tissue engineering. *Progress in Polymer Science* 36: 238–268.

Kruegel, J., and N. Miosge. 2010. Basement membrane components are key players in specialized extracellular matrices. *Cellular and Molecular Life Science* 67 (17): 2879–2895.

Miranti, C. K., and J. S. Brugge. 2002. Sensing the environment: A historical perspective on integrin signal transduction. *Nature Cell Biology* 4 (4): E83–E90.

Pardi, R. 2010. Signal transduction by adhesion receptors. *Nature Education* 3 (9): 38.

Chapter 9

Dynamic versus Static Seeding of Cells onto Biomaterial Scaffolds

9.1 Background

Cell seeding onto a biomaterial scaffold is commonly an initial step in tissue engineering. A successful cell-seeding strategy achieves a high seeding efficiency to avoid wasting cells, short inoculation periods, and a high density and uniform distribution of cells within the scaffold (Vunjak-Novakovic et al. 1998). Many different methods have been developed to achieve these goals; however, the specific approach depends on a number of factors, including cell and scaffold type, size, and shape.

Scaffolds used for tissue engineering include both biologic and synthetic materials. Some common biologic materials include decellularized extracellular matrix and purified natural polymers such as collagen and fibrin. Common synthetic materials for tissue engineering include polylactic acid, polyglycolic acid, and their copolymers. Despite the diversity of scaffolds in use, there are very few off-the-shelf commercially available scaffolds. Those that do exist are expensive and are limited in their geometry and composition.

Ultrafoam® is a bovine collagen sponge produced by Davol and marketed as a topical hemostatic. In its intended use, the collagen acts as a framework to facilitate clot formation. Ultrafoam's biocompatibility, high surface-to-volume ratio, demonstrated adhesive properties, and wide availability make it a potentially useful scaffold for tissue engineering. Ultrafoam has been used experimentally as a scaffold for bone tissue engineering (Meinel et al. 2004); however, the efficiency of cell attachment to Ultrafoam in tissue-engineering applications has not been reported.

9.2 Learning Objectives

The objectives of this experiment are to

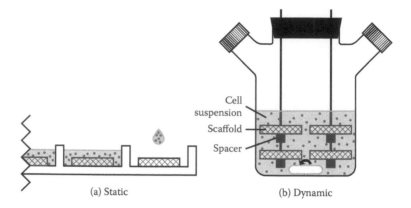

Figure 9.1

Schematic of the static and dynamic methods for seeding cells onto a biomaterial scaffold. (a) In the static method, a suspension of cells is seeded directly onto the top surface of a scaffold within a standard culture vessel. (b) In the dynamic method, scaffolds are suspended in a spinner flask. The flask continuously stirs a suspension of cells around the scaffolds with the goal of cells attaching to the interior pores of the scaffold.

- Investigate the potential use of Ultrafoam as a tissue-engineering scaffold
- Measure the efficiency of cell attachment for two different methods of seeding cells on Ultrafoam scaffolds: static seeding in a multiwell plate (Figure 9.1a) and dynamic seeding using a spinner flask (Figure 9.1b)
- Using statistics, compare the effectiveness of the two different seeding methods
- Learn to perform a widely applicable DNA assay using a fluorometer

9.3 Overview of Experiment

The overall procedure for this experiment involves seeding a suspension of fibroblasts onto a collagen scaffold overnight (or longer) and then determining the number and percentage of cells that attached to the scaffold. The scaffolds will be prepared by punching cores out of a sheet of Ultrafoam collagen sponge. Two different seeding methods will be compared to determine which results in the highest seeding efficiency: static seeding in a multiwell plate or dynamic seeding using a spinner flask ($n = 4$). To quantify the number of cells attached within the Ultrafoam scaffold, the scaffold and cells will be enzymatically digested; mixed with a fluorescent DNA-binding dye, PicoGreen®; and the fluorescence intensity measured using a fluorometer. A calibration curve will be generated from a range of DNA standards to relate fluorescence intensity to DNA concentration.

9.4 Safety Notes

According to the manufacturer, the mutagenicity and toxicity of PicoGreen have not been assessed. Because this reagent binds to nucleic acids, it should be treated as a potential mutagen, handled with care, and disposed of in accordance with local regulations. Use good lab practices and review all relevant MSDSs.

9.5 Materials

In addition to the general equipment and supplies, the following are needed to complete this experiment:

9.5.1 Reagents and Consumables

- $>10 \times 10^6$ 3T3 Cells in culture (e.g., 3–4 × 100 mm confluent dishes)
- 1.2 cm Sterile biopsy punch
- Ultrafoam collagen sponge (≥ 15 cm^2)
- 3T3 Media (recipe follows)
- 0.25% Trypsin with EDTA (1X)
- Trypan blue
- Phosphate-buffered EDTA (PBE)
- 50X Proteinase-K (25 mg/mL in PBE)
- PicoGreen dsDNA assay kit (including TE buffer and 100 µg/mL DNA standard; Molecular Probes)

9.5.2 Equipment and Supplies

- Sterile spinner flask assembly
- Sterile spacers
- Sterile forceps
- Sterile stir bar
- Promega quanti-fluor fluorometer (EX: 480 nm, EM: 520 nm) with minicell cuvettes

9.6 Recipes

3T3 Media. Add 50 mL bovine calf serum (BCS) and 5 mL of 100X penicillin/streptomycin (P/S) to 445 mL of DMEM (high glucose).

0.1 *M* Phosphate buffer. Reconstitute according to manufacturer's instructions or purchase 1X solution.

PBE. Dissolve ethylenediaminetetraacetic acid disodium salt dihydrate (EDTA, MW = 372) at 1.86 mg/mL in 0.1 *M* phosphate buffer, adjust pH to 7.1 with HCl and NaOH, and store at room temperature.

50X Proteinase-K stock. Dilute proteinase-K in PBE to a concentration of 25 mg/mL, prepare 100 µL aliquots, and store at –20°C for up to a year. This is a 50X stock solution. Dilute the stock in PBE as needed.

1X TE buffer. Dilute the 20X TE buffer supplied with the PicoGreen kit in deionized water (dH₂O).

100 µg/mL DNA standard. Prepare 5 µL aliquots of the DNA standard provided with the PicoGreen kit. Store at –20°C.

PicoGreen. Prepare 5 µL aliquots of the 200X solution provided with the PicoGreen kit. Store at –20°C.

9.7 Methods

9.7.1 Session 1: Prepare Scaffolds

1. Prepare the biosafety cabinet (BSC) for use by wiping it down with 70% ethanol and arranging necessary reagents and disposables.

2. Prepare the scaffolds: Working on a sterile surface, such as a petri dish, use a sterile biopsy punch to cut eight scaffolds out of the sheet of Ultrafoam. Estimate the thickness of the scaffolds.

3. Arrange the scaffolds for the static seeding condition:
   a. Using sterile forceps, place four of the scaffolds into individual wells of a 24-well tissue culture plate.
   b. Set the 24-well plate aside within the BSC.

4. Assemble the spinner flasks for the dynamic seeding condition:
   a. Carefully open the autoclave pouch containing the spinner flask.
   b. Working on the sterile surface of the pouch or a spare petri dish, use forceps to thread the remaining four scaffolds gently onto the cap assembly, including a spacer between each pair of scaffolds (Figure 9.1b).
   c. Place a sterile stir bar in the bottom of the spinner flask.
   d. Tightly attach the cap assembly, with scaffolds, to the spinner flask.
   e. Set the spinner flask aside within the BSC.

9.7.2 Session 2: Seed Cells

1. In a 37°C water bath, warm 3T3 media and ~15 mL of trypsin.

2. Prepare the BSC for use by wiping it down with 70% ethanol and arranging necessary reagents and disposables.

3. Hydrate the scaffolds:
   a. Gently add 46 mL of 3T3 media to the spinner flask through one of the side ports.
   b. Add 1 mL of 3T3 media to each of the scaffolds in the multiwell plate.

4. Prepare 3T3 cells for seeding:

   a. Remove the 3T3 cells from the incubator.

   b. View the cells under the microscope. Note the cell morphology and extent of confluence.

   c. Trypsinize the cells (refer to trypsinization protocol in Appendix 1).

   d. Resuspend the cells in 5 mL of 3T3 media.

   e. Count the cells using a hemacytometer (refer to hemacytometer protocol in Appendix 2).

   f. Dilute the suspension to a final concentration of 1×10^6 cells/mL.

   g. Collect a 250 μL sample of your cell suspension in a vial with a threaded cap (e.g., cryovial) labeled "Seeding Suspension." Store this sample in a –20°C freezer for future use.

5. Seed the cells onto the scaffolds (static and dynamic conditions):

   a. Mix the cell suspension thoroughly and add 1 mL to each scaffold within the 24-well plate.

   b. Place the 24-well plate in the incubator.

   c. Add 4 mL of the cell suspension to the spinner flask through a side port.

   d. Cap the side ports tightly and then loosen the caps approximately half a turn to allow gas exchange between the flask and the surroundings.

   e. Lightly spray a magnetic stir plate with 70% ethanol and place it on the bottom shelf of the incubator. Connect the power cord. Place the spinner flask on the stir plate and adjust the speed to achieve ~50 revolutions per minute. If it is necessary to run the power cord through the incubator's front door, be sure the door is closed tightly and the temperature and percentage of CO_2 are stable.

9.7.3 Session 3: Digest Cell-Seeded Scaffolds and Cell Suspensions

1. After 18–48 h, remove the spinner flask and 24-well plate from the incubator.

2. Carefully remove each scaffold from the cap assembly and place each one into a labeled cryovial. Repeat for the scaffolds in the 24-well plate.

3. Warm a water bath to 50°C.

4. Make a 0.5 mg/mL proteinase-K solution by combining 100 μL of the 50X (25 mg/mL) stock solution with 4.9 mL PBE.

5. Add 250 μL proteinase-K into each cryovial containing a scaffold or sample of the cell seeding suspension collected during Session 2. Make sure the tissue is completely immersed in the digest solution. Cap the cryovial so that the solution does not evaporate.

6. Place vial or tube in the 50°C water bath and wait at least 8 h for complete digestion. Be careful that the water level is low enough (or that the rack is on a "lift") so that the vials or tubs are not fully submersed.

7. After digestion, the samples can be stored in the freezer until you are ready to perform the PicoGreen DNA assay.

9.7.4 Session 4: Quantify Cell Attachment

1. Turn on and configure the fluorometer to excite at ~480 nm and measure emission at ~520 nm.

2. Remove two 5 µL PicoGreen aliquots, the DNA standards, and the samples (seeding suspension, static and dynamic scaffolds) from the freezer and allow them to thaw.

3. Prepare the PicoGreen dye solution as described in the PicoGreen protocol (Appendix 3).

4. Prepare the DNA standards (200–0 ng DNA/mL final volume) as described in the PicoGreen protocol.

5. Generate a standard curve as described in the PicoGreen protocol. If the standard curve is not linear, try to identify the source of error and repeat until a reliable standard curve is obtained.

6. Prepare duplicate samples as described in the PicoGreen protocol. For this particular experiment, mixing 25 µL of each sample with 225 µL TE buffer should yield a concentration within the range of the standards. *Note: It is very important to vortex each sample before and after diluting it.*

7. Perform the PicoGreen assay to measure the DNA concentration in each sample. If any sample is out of range of the standards or the fluorometer detection limit, dilute the sample more and repeat the measurement until the reading falls within the working range of the calibration curve. Make careful notes regarding the dilutions in your lab notebook.

9.8 Data Processing and Reporting

Briefly report the results of your experiment in paragraph and graphical form. Each of the key results to report in text, figure, and/or table format is described next.

1. Include a graph of the DNA standard curve (x-axis: DNA concentration, y-axis: fluorescence). Display the equation of the best-fit line and the corresponding r^2 value on the graph.

2. Include a table, similar to Table 9.1, displaying the raw data and subsequent calculations from the PicoGreen assay. Briefly describe each calculation in the text. *Note: The DNA content of a 3T3 cell is 13.7 pg/cell* (Patterson 1979).

3. From the DNA content of your samples, calculate the *total number of cells that attached* to each scaffold. Generate a bar graph displaying the average number of cells that attached to the scaffolds for each seeding method (static or dynamic). Include error bars corresponding to the standard deviation (SD).

4. From the DNA content of your samples and the seeding suspension, calculate the *percentage of seeded cells that attached to each scaffold*. (For dynamic, assume exactly one-fourth of the cells in the cell suspension were available to attach to each scaffold.) Generate a bar graph that displays the average percentage of cells that attached to the scaffolds for each seeding method (static or dynamic). Include error bars corresponding to the SD.

TABLE 9.1
Suggested Format for Reporting Data Collected from the DNA Assay

	Sample Description			
	Sample of Cell Suspension	Dynamic 1	Dynamic 2	...
Fluorescence				...
Fluorescence of duplicate				...
Mean fluorescence				...
Percentage difference in duplicates				
[DNA] in cuvette (picograms/milliliter)[a]				...
Dilution factor[b]				...
[DNA] in sample (picograms/milliliter)				...
[Cells] in sample (cells/milliliter)				...
Total cells in sample				...

[a] Calculate from the average fluorescence and the standard curve.
[b] Dilution factor = total volume in cuvette ÷ volume of undiluted sample in cuvette.

5. The density of the seeding suspension (in cells per milliliter) was originally determined by hemacytometer counting. A sample of the seeding suspension was later analyzed using a DNA assay and the density of the seeding suspension was determined by this alternate method. Report on the agreement or disagreement of these two methods and identify possible sources of error.

6. Statistical analysis: use a t-test to determine if seeding method (static vs. dynamic) significantly affected the number of attached cells. Report the degrees of freedom, critical t-value corresponding to $p < 0.05$, the p-value obtained from your data, and the statistical power.

9.9 Prelab Questions

1. Why is optimizing cell seeding efficiency (percentage of seeded cells that attach) important for commercial tissue engineering? Present your answer in terms of product efficacy, cost, and manufacturing.

2. What seeding method do you think will result in the highest seeding efficiency? Explain why you believe this method will produce a higher seeding efficiency than the other method.

3. In addition to seeding efficiency, what are some other differences that may result from the use of the different seeding methods? Briefly describe one experiment to determine if one or more of these differences exist.

4. Imagine this is the first in a series of experiments you will conduct to develop a tissue-engineered ligament. Identify five qualitative design goals and five corresponding quantitative specifications for the tissue-engineered ligament.

9.10 Postlab Questions

1. Approximate the cell density within the scaffolds after seeding. How does this compare to the cell density within human tissues? Is having a particular number of cells initially seeded critical? Why or why not?

2. If you were to repeat the experiment again, what modifications would you make?

3. Discuss possible modifications that could be made to the scaffold to improve efficiency of cell attachment.

4. Compare and contrast this experiment's methods and results with those reported in Vunjak-Novakovic and colleagues (1998). How were our methods similar? Different? How might these differences affect the results?

References

Meinel, L., V. Karageorgiou, S. Hofmann, R. Fajardo, B. Snyder, C. Li, L. Zichner, R. Langer, G. Vunjak-Novakovic, and D. L. Kaplan. 2004. Engineering bone-like tissue in vitro using human bone marrow stem cells and silk scaffolds. *Journal of Biomedical Materials Research A* 71 (1): 25–34.

Patterson, M. K., Jr. 1979. Measurement of growth and viability of cells in culture. In *Methods in enzymology,* eds. S. P. Colowick, N. O. Kaplan, and W. B. Jakoby. New York: Academic Press.

Vunjak-Novakovic, G., B. Obradovic, I. Martin, P. M. Bursac, R. Langer, and L. E. Freed. 1998. Dynamic cell seeding of polymer scaffolds for cartilage tissue engineering. *Biotechnology Progress* 14 (2): 193–202.

Chapter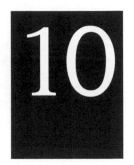

Cell Patterning Using Microcontact Printing

10.1 Background

Cell patterning refers to the ability to direct cell adhesion with high spatial precision. It is a useful tool for both clinical and research applications of tissue engineering. For example, to manufacture a complex engineered tissue, it may be necessary to control the spatial arrangement of cells within the tissue or to tightly regulate cell–cell and cell–matrix interaction. As a research tool, cell patterning can be used to investigate the role of cell–cell and cell–matrix interactions in regulating various cellular functions.

Cell patterning in two dimensions is achieved by seeding a suspension of anchorage-dependent cells onto a substrate containing adhesive extracellular matrix (ECM) "islands" to which the cells preferentially attach. Two methods are commonly used to create the adhesive islands: microfluidic patterning and microcontact printing (μCP). In microfluidic patterning, a solution of an ECM protein or other adhesive molecule is forced through a series of very small channels and then allowed to settle, in a pattern, onto the substrate. Microcontact printing uses a stamp, custom fabricated from a soft polymer, to transfer an adhesive protein or intermediary directly onto the substrate (James et al. 1998; Bernard et al. 1998; Singhvi et al. 1994). This process is analogous to using a traditional stamp to transfer a pattern of ink onto a sheet of paper (Figure 10.1). In this experiment, you will use laminin, a major constituent of the basement membrane, as the adhesive "ink."

The stamps used for μCP are fabricated using a process called soft lithography, which is described in detail in Appendix 5. Briefly, an elastic polymer is poured over a template (also called a master), cured, and then removed to yield a "rubber stamp" with a topography that is the exact negative of the master's. The most frequently used polymer for biomedical applications of soft lithography is polydimethylsiloxane (PDMS). PDMS is a good choice for biomedical applications because it is optically clear, gas permeable, flexible, and biocompatible (Weibel, Diluzio, and Whitesides 2007; Lee et al. 2004). The features on the master, the stamp, and the patterned surface typically have dimensions of microns. To achieve this spatial resolution, a

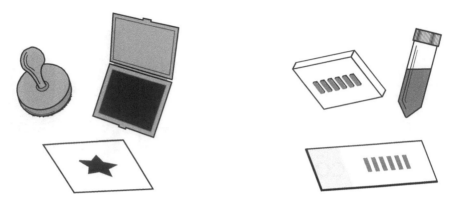

Figure 10.1
A rubber stamp is used to transfer ink from an inkpad onto a piece of paper. Analogously, a PDMS stamp is used to transfer an adhesive protein from an aqueous solution onto a culture surface, such as a glass slide.

master is fabricated using a silicon wafer with techniques originally developed for the electronics industry. For the purpose of demonstrating μCP, any object with a millimeter- or micron-scale, three-dimensional patterned surface can be used to cast a PDMS stamp.

Microcontact printing has been used extensively as an experimental tool to study cell growth (Chen et al. 1997; Singhvi et al. 1994), apoptosis (Chen et al. 1997), differentiation (McBeath et al. 2004), and maintenance of cell phenotype (Singhvi et al. 1994). For example, Chen and colleagues patterned substrates with fibronectin islands of various sizes to control endothelial cell spreading either within a single island (Figure 10.2a and b) or across multiple, smaller islands (Figure 10.2c). Using this approach, they demonstrated that the extent of cell spreading determined whether a cell underwent proliferation or apoptosis in a manner that was independent of the total contact area between the cell and the underlying fibronectin.

Differentiation of human mesenchymal stem cells (MSCs) is also controlled by cell shape (McBeath et al. 2004). Specifically, MSCs allowed to spread have more similarity with bone cells while those restricted to a round morphology have more similarity with fat cells (McBeath et al. 2004). Similarly, liver cells, called hepatocytes, maintained their tissue-specific function of secreting albumin when cultured on small adhesive islands (40 × 40 μm) but not when cultured on unpatterned substrates or large adhesive islands (100 × 100 μm) (Singhvi et al. 1994).

Muscle is an example of a tissue that may require precise control of cell arrangement to engineer a functional tissue. Proper skeletal and heart muscle function relies on the parallel arrangement of muscle fibers. These fibers form when multiple, immature myoblasts fuse together to form multinucleated myotubes. Patterning of myoblast or cardiac muscle cells has been explored as a method for influencing in vitro muscle engineering (Molnar et al. 2007; McDevitt et al. 2002). In this experiment, you will pattern a common murine skeletal myoblast cell line, C2C12, on a microcontact printed laminin substrate.

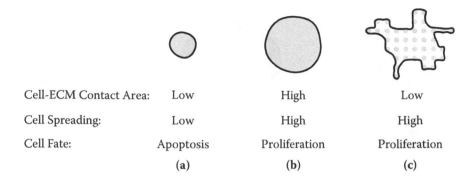

Cell-ECM Contact Area:	Low	High	Low
Cell Spreading:	Low	High	High
Cell Fate:	Apoptosis	Proliferation	Proliferation
	(a)	**(b)**	**(c)**

Figure 10.2
Endothelial cells (outlined in black) that were confined to small fibronectin islands (shaded regions) underwent apoptosis (a), while those that were allowed to spread on large islands (b) or across multiple small islands (c) proliferated. The total contact area between the cell and underlying fibronectin was the same in (a) and (c), indicating that shape, not total cell–matrix contact area, was the predominant influence. (From Chen et al. 1997. *Science* 276: 1425–1428.)

10.2 Learning Objectives

The objectives of this experiment are to

- Fabricate reusable PDMS stamps for μCP of proteins
- Reproducibly pattern fluorescently labeled laminin in a culture dish
- Determine whether C2C12 cells preferentially adhere to and spread on the patterned substrate
- Using statistics, test if a single stamp can be used to produce multiple stamped patterns of similar quality without "re-inking" the stamp

10.3 Overview of Experiment

Microcontact printing will be used to generate a defined pattern of C2C12 cells. The first step in the experiment is to fabricate a stamp by curing PDMS on a template or "master." An American penny will be used as a master in this experiment because the columns of the Lincoln Memorial make a convenient linear pattern on which to grow the cells. After polymerization, the stamp is removed from the master and "inked" with laminin. The laminin is then stamped onto a multiwell plate pretreated with Pluronic® F-127, a block polymer of polyethylene glycol–polypropylene glycol–polyethylene glycol that renders the nonprinted region of the culture substrate nonadhesive. The laminin has been labeled with a fluorescent dye, Cy3 (EX: 550 nm, EM: 570 nm) so that the pattern can be visualized using fluorescence microscopy (Figure 10.3a).

Next, you will seed C2C12 cells on the patterned laminin surface, allow the cells to attach (Figure 10.3b), wash away nonadherent cells, and maintain the cells in

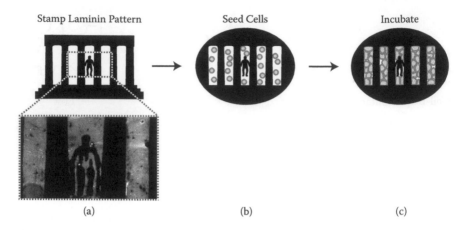

Figure 10.3
Schematic overview of the patterning experiment. (a) Laminin is stamped onto a tissue culture substrate in the pattern of a penny. The laminin pattern appears light against a dark background, when visualized using fluorescence microscopy, because the laminin is fluorescently labeled. (b) Cells are seeded and adhere to the laminin-stamped regions. (c) With time in culture, the adherent cells spread on the laminin pattern and proliferate.

culture so that they spread on the laminin pattern (Figure 10.3c). In the final session of this experiment, you will label the patterned cells with a fluorescent cytoplasmic dye, called CMFDA (EX: 492 nm, EM: 517 nm), and acquire fluorescent micrographs of the patterned cells and underlying laminin.

10.4 Safety Notes

Use good lab practices and review all relevant MSDSs.

10.5 Materials

In addition to the general equipment and supplies, the following are needed to complete this experiment:

10.5.1 Reagents and Consumables

- Sylgard® 184 (PDMS)
- Three American pennies
- Non-tissue-culture-treated 12-well plate
- 1X Phosphate-buffered saline (PBS)

- 0.2% Pluronic F-127 in PBS
- ~1 mg/mL Cy3-Labeled laminin (EX: 550 nm, EM: 570 nm)
- >3 × 10^6 C2C12 cells in monolayer culture (e.g., 2 × 100 mm confluent dishes)
- C2C12 Media (recipe follows)
- 1X PBS + 1% penicillin/streptomycin (PBS + P/S)
- Serum-free media (recipe follows)
- 0.25% Trypsin with EDTA (1X)
- Trypan blue
- 1.2 cm Sterile biopsy punch
- 10 mM CellTracker™ green (CMFDA, EX: 492 nm, EM: 517 nm)

10.5.2 Equipment and Supplies

- House or compressed nitrogen or air
- Vacuum desiccator
- Lab oven (optional)
- Microscope equipped for fluorescence and digital imaging (A dual emission filter for simultaneously viewing CMFDA [EX: 492 nm, EM: 517 nm] and Cy3 [EX: 550 nm, EM: 570 nm] is suggested.)

10.6 Recipes

1 mg/mL Cy3-Labeled laminin. Prior to use, the instructor will label laminin with Cy3, a fluorescent dye compatible with most rhodamine filter sets. Store Cy3–laminin at –20°C at ~1 mg/mL in 30 μL aliquots.

0.2% Pluronic F-127. Dissolve 0.1 g of Pluronic in 50 mL of PBS, filter-sterilize, and store at room temperature (RT).

C2C12 media. Add 50 mL bovine calf serum (BCS) and 5 mL of 100X penicillin/streptomycin (P/S) to 445 mL of DMEM (high glucose).

5% BSA stock. Dissolve 0.5 g of BSA in 10 mL of PBS. Gently mix by rocking at 4°C. Once it is dissolved, sterile-filter using a 0.2 μm syringe filter and store at 4°C. Do not use stored solution if residual, nondissolved BSA is visible by eye.

Serum-free media. Add 2 mL of 5% BSA stock and 1 mL P/S for every 100 mL DMEM (high glucose).

CMFDA. Dilute CMFDA, as supplied, to 10 mM in sterile DMSO. Store 10 μL aliquots at –20°C.

1X PBS. Add 50 mL 10X PBS (with Ca^{2+} and Mg^{2+}) to 400 mL deionized H_2O (dH_2O). Mix well, adjust pH to 7.4 with HCl and NaOH, bring total volume to 500 mL with dH_2O, and either sterile-filter through a 0.2 μm filter or autoclave.

PBS + P/S. Add 1 mL of P/S for every 99 mL PBS.

10.7 Methods

10.7.1 Session 1: Fabricate the PDMS Stamps

1. Clean the pennies:
   a. Thoroughly wash with soap, water, and a scouring pad.
   b. Rinse with water followed by 70% ethanol.
   c. Remove any loose dirt from the surface using a stream of nitrogen or air.
2. Place the pennies, Lincoln Memorial side up, in separate petri dishes or far from each other in one dish.
3. Calculate the volume of PDMS needed based on the surface area of the dishes and knowing that the PDMS should be poured to create an ~3 mm high layer. Make ~200% of what is needed to account for volume loss during pipetting due to the high viscosity of the PDMS.
4. In a disposable 50 mL centrifuge tube, combine the PDMS and curing agents in a 10:1 weight-to-weight ratio (w/w) and *mix thoroughly* using a pipette or disposable utensil.
5. Centrifuge the PDMS for 5 min at 500 g to remove any air bubbles.
6. Gently pour the PDMS over the masters to reach a height of ~3 mm.
7. Place the dishes in a vacuum desiccator and apply vacuum for 30 min (or longer as needed to remove air bubbles). If necessary, it is acceptable to stack multiple dishes within the desiccator.
8. Remove the dishes from the vacuum desiccator and cure the PDMS in a 60°C oven for at least 4 h or for >48 hrs at RT.

10.7.2 Session 2: Microcontact Print the Laminin

1. Prepare the biosafety cabinet (BSC) for use by wiping it down with 70% ethanol and arranging necessary reagents and disposables.
2. In the BSC, pretreat a sterile, non-tissue-culture-treated 12-well plate with Pluronic F-127:
   a. Add 1 mL of sterile Pluronic solution to two wells in each of the first three rows of the plate (six wells total). Label the wells so that you know which have been pretreated.
   b. Allow the Pluronic to adsorb to the surface while you prepare the stamps as described next (≥30 min). Record the time in your lab notebook.

Steps 3–6 and 8 do not need to be performed sterilely.

3. Gently peel the PDMS off the masters.
4. Use a biopsy punch to remove the surrounding PDMS from the patterned regions. Keep the stamping surface clean and handle the stamps only with forceps for the remainder of the experiment.

5. Verify that the stamps contain the desired pattern either by visual inspection or by viewing them using transmitted light microscopy.

6. "Ink" the stamps:

   a. Place the stamps, patterned side up, in a clean petri dish. Press the stamps down firmly so that they stick to the dish.

   b. Remove the stock 1 mg/mL laminin from the freezer and *slowly* bring it to RT.

   c. Dilute to 30 µg/mL in PBS and mix well with a pipette.

   d. Pipette a small amount (~200 µL/cm^2) of the laminin solution on the patterned side of the PDMS stamps, gently spread the drop with the pipette tip so that the entire pattern is covered, and allow the protein to be adsorbed for 30 min at RT while protecting from light. Record the time in your lab notebook.

7. Return to the BSC to rinse the Pluronic-treated wells:

   a. If it has been at least 30 min since adding Pluronic to the well plate, aspirate the Pluronic solution and rinse each well twice with 4 mL of sterile PBS + PS.

   b. After the final rinse, aspirate all the liquid out of the wells and allow them to dry completely in the BSC. Leave the lid off the plate while the wells are drying.

8. Dry the laminin-coated stamps:

   a. After incubating the stamps with laminin for 30 min (as described in Step 6d), use a lab tissue to wick off excess solution from the stamps, being careful not to touch the patterned region.

   b. Thoroughly dry the PDMS stamps under a stream of nitrogen or air. *Note: The easiest method for drying the stamps is to leave them stuck to the dish and flow nitrogen or air over the whole dish.*

9. Return to the BSC to stamp the laminin onto the multiwell plate:

   a. Using sterile forceps, place each stamp (patterned side down) into one of the Pluoronic-treated wells. Press down firmly using an upside down, capped microfuge tube to bring the stamps in close contact with the surface.

   b. Allow the stamps to remain in contact for 1 min without moving them *at all.*

   c. Repeat with a second well so that each stamp is used twice. Do not re-ink with laminin between stamps. Keep track of which wells were stamped first and which were stamped second.

   d. Add 0.5 mL of sterile PBS + PS to each well.

10. Set up the microscope for fluorescence imaging; use a filter cube compatible with Cy3 (EX: 550 nm, EM: 570 nm). Allow the lamp to warm up for ~15 min.

11. View the printed wells using a microscope equipped for fluorescence to verify that the laminin was printed in the desired pattern. Note any differences between stamp replicates in your lab notebook. If significant variability exists, capture representative digital images to document these differences. If not, capture several images to document the typical quality of the patterns. *Note: Exposure of the samples to the fluorescent lamp should be minimized to avoid photobleaching, which is the destruction of the dye resulting in diminished brightness.*

12. Obtain a calibration image so that you will be able to add a scale bar to representative micrographs when documenting your results. You may get a calibration image from

your instructor or acquire an image of a stage micrometer or hemacytometer grid using the same magnification as in the micrographs.

13. Wrap the plates with foil to protect them from light and store them at 4°C until session 3.

10.7.3 Session 3: Pattern the Cells

1. In a 37°C water bath, warm ~25 mL of C2C12 media, ~15 mL of serum-free media (DMEM + 0.1% BSA + P/S), and ~8 mL of trypsin.

2. Prepare the BSC for use by wiping it down with 70% ethanol and arranging necessary reagents and disposables.

3. Prepare the C2C12 cells for seeding:
   a. Remove the cells from the incubator.
   b. View the cells under the microscope. Note the cell morphology and extent of confluence.
   c. Trypsinize the cells (refer to trypsinization protocol in Appendix 1), rinse once in media, and once in serum-free media.
   d. Resuspend the cells in 1 mL of serum-free media.
   e. Count the cells using a hemacytometer (refer to hemacytometer protocol in Appendix 2).
   f. Dilute the suspension to a final concentration of 1×10^6 cells/mL in serum-free media. You will need at least 3 mL of the cell suspension at this concentration.

4. Retrieve your stamped dish and aspirate the PBS + 1% P/S.

5. Pipette 0.5 mL of the 1×10^6 cells/mL suspension into each of the six wells containing replicate laminin patterns.

6. Allow the cells to attach in the incubator for at least 45 min.

7. Check the cells under the microscope to verify that they have settled and attached to the patterned surface. If not, incubate the cells ~15 min longer before proceeding to the next step.

8. Gently aspirate off the media and rinse the wells with 1 mL C2C12 media to remove any cells that did not adhere.

9. Gently add 1 mL C2C12 media to each well and return the plate to the incubator. Culture the cells 2 days or longer to allow the adherent cells to spread and proliferate on the laminin surface. For long-term cultures, change the media every 2–3 days.

10.7.4 Session 4: Image the Patterned Cells

1. In a 37°C water bath, warm 10 mL of PBS and 10 mL of C2C12 media.

2. Prepare the BSC for use by wiping it down with 70% ethanol and arranging necessary reagents and disposables.

3. Dilute 10 μL of the stock 10 mM CMFDA with 10 mL of PBS for a final concentration of 10 μM. Add 1 mL to each well of patterned cells and incubate for 15 min at 37°C.

4. Replace the CMFDA solution with warm C2C12 media.

5. Set up the microscope for fluorescence imaging; use a filter cube or cubes compatible with Cy3 (EX: 550 nm, EM: 570 nm) and CMFDA (EX: 492 nm, EM: 517 nm). Allow the lamp to warm up for ~15 min. View the patterned cells using a low-powered objective.

6. Capture representative digital pictures showing the pattern of laminin and pattern of cells for each well. Depending on the fluorescent filter sets available, it may be necessary to take two separate images (one of laminin and one of cells) and then overlay them for analysis.

7. Obtain a calibration image at this magnification so that you will be able to add a scale bar to representative micrographs when documenting your results.

10.8 Data Processing and Reporting

Briefly report the results of your experiment. The key figures to include in your report, poster, or abstract are described next.

1. Use image processing software, such as ImageJ, to characterize the *quality* of each laminin pattern and report these results. Each research team must determine a meaningful outcome measure to characterize pattern quality and must justify the approach used.

2. Describe any variability in the quality of the laminin patterns. Discuss possible sources of this variability and whether the observed variability appears to be a result of random or systematic error. Include representative micrographs to illustrate any differences or, if no significant differences exist, a typical pattern.

3. Statistical analysis: determine if using a stamp multiple times without re-inking significantly affects laminin pattern quality under the conditions used here. Report the statistical test used, p-value obtained from your data, and statistical power. *Note: The appropriate statistical test depends on the outcome measure used in step 1.*

4. In one professional-quality figure with six panels, include representative micrographs of each pattern of cells. Include a scale bar. Summarize your observations within the text.

10.9 Prelab Questions

1. What other adhesive proteins or peptides could be used in this experiment instead of laminin? Provide justification.

2.

   a. Which class of cell surface receptors is responsible for the adhesion of C2C12 cells to the laminin substrate? Which specific member(s) of this class of receptors is (are) likely involved?

   b. Briefly describe an experiment you could perform to test your hypothesis.

3. Review the paper by Tan and colleagues (2004) when formulating your answer to the following:

a. What property of an untreated polystyrene surface is preferable to a tissue-culture-treated polystyrene surface for patterning using the protocol outlined in this lab? Briefly explain.

b. What quantitative measure is used to characterize this property?

4.

a. Identify another example of an engineered tissue that would require a precise arrangement (or geometric control) of one or more cell types. Describe and sketch the organization of the native tissue; include labels for different cell types and extracellular matrix components. Briefly explain the significance of cell arrangement within the tissue to the tissue's function.

b. Identify and briefly describe one functional limitation of μCP for large-scale production of engineered tissues.

10.10 Postlab Questions

1. Molnar et al. (2007) reported that differentiation of C2C12 cells into myoblasts depends on the dimensions of the protein pattern. Specifically, patterned lines 30 μm wide were optimal for supporting the formation of single myotubes. Cells cultured on lines 50 μm wide formed multiple myotubes while those cultured on lines below 10 μm did not form myotubes.

a. Estimate or measure the characteristic length of the pattern used in this experiment and compare it to the patterns used in Molnar et al.

b. How would you expect the cells in this experiment to organize if maintained in culture for a longer period of time? Justify your answer.

c. How do the dimensions of a mature mouse myocyte *in vivo* compare to the protein patterns used in this experiment and in those reported by Molnar et al.? Cite your source and comment on the significance of this finding.

d. What would be the functional consequence of randomly aligned muscle fibers in a tissue-engineered medical product?

2. If you were to repeat the experiment again what modifications would you make? Why?

3. Write a detailed protocol that could be used to differentiate the patterned myoblasts and assess the organization of actin and/or myosin into myofibrils. Include references to related studies published in the literature.

References

Bernard, A., E. Delamarche, H. Schmid, B. Michel, H. R. Bosshard, and H. Biebuyck. 1998. Printing patterns of proteins. *Langmuir* 14 (9): 2225–2229.

Chen, C. S., M. Mrksich, S. Huang, G. M. Whitesides, and D. E. Ingber. 1997. Geometric control of cell life and death. *Science* 276 (5317): 1425–1428.

James, C. D., R. C. Davis, L. Kam, H. G. Craighead, M. Isaacson, J. N. Turner, and W. Shain. 1998. Patterned protein layers on solid substrates by thin stamp microcontact printing. *Langmuir* 14 (4): 741–744.

Lee, J. N., X. Jiang, D. Ryan, and G. M. Whitesides. 2004. Compatibility of mammalian cells on surfaces of poly(dimethylsiloxane). *Langmuir* 20 (26): 11684–11691.

McBeath, R., D. M. Pirone, C. M. Nelson, K. Bhadriraju, and C. S. Chen. 2004. Cell shape, cytoskeletal tension, and RhoA regulate stem cell lineage commitment. *Developmental Cell* 6 (4): 483–495.

McDevitt, T. C., J. C. Angello, M. L. Whitney, H. Reinecke, S. D. Hauschka, C. E. Murry, and P. S. Stayton. 2002. In vitro generation of differentiated cardiac myofibers on micropatterned laminin surfaces. *Journal of Biomedical Materials Research* 60 (3): 472–479.

Molnar, P., W. Wang, A. Natarajan, J. W. Rumsey, and J. J. Hickman. 2007. Photolithographic patterning of C2C12 myotubes using vitronectin as growth substrate in serum-free medium. *Biotechnology Progress* 23 (1): 265–268.

Singhvi, R., A. Kumar, G. P. Lopez, G. N. Stephanopoulos, D. I. Wang, G. M. Whitesides, and D. E. Ingber. 1994. Engineering cell shape and function. *Science* 264 (5159): 696–698.

Tan, J. L., W. Liu, C. M. Nelson, S. Raghavan, and C. S. Chen. 2004. Simple approach to micropattern cells on common culture substrates by tuning substrate wettability. *Tissue Engineering* 10 (5–6): 865–872.

Weibel, D. B., W. R. Diluzio, and G. M. Whitesides. 2007. Microfabrication meets microbiology. *Nature Reviews Microbiology* 5 (3): 209–218.

Chapter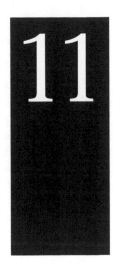

Measuring and Modeling the Motility of a Cell Population Using an Under-Agarose Assay

11.1 Background

After implantation of a tissue-engineered medical product (TEMP), the body will undergo a wound-healing response, ideally leading to full integration of the implant with the native tissue. Controlling migration of cells during wound healing provides a mechanism for influencing the remodeling and eventual integration of the TEMP. Many TEMPs require a blood supply for long-term survival after implantation. During angiogenesis, cells migrate from the surrounding tissue into the TEMP in order to establish a blood vessel network throughout the tissue. Finally, the migration of cells from the TEMP into the surrounding area may be a functional requirement for the success of the implant. For these reasons, understanding and controlling cell migration is important for tissue engineering.

11.1.1 Signals That Direct Cell Migration

Chemokines are a class of proteins that induce and direct cell migration. Chemotaxis refers to the migration of cells in a direction determined by a gradient of a diffusible chemical, such as a chemokine. Cells are attracted to and migrate toward the source of a chemokine; thus, chemokines function as chemoattractants. When present in a uniform concentration in the environment (i.e., no gradient), chemokines affect the speed, but not the direction, of cell migration. Stimulation of migration in random directions in this manner is called chemokinesis. Nondiffusible signals on the extracellular matrix or the surface of neighboring cells can also direct cell migration. The effect of a chemokine or other signals on the migration of a specific cell type can be studied using in vitro assays.

11.1.2 In Vitro Migration Assays

There are several popular assays for studying cell migration, including Boyden chambers, Zigmond chambers, and under-agarose assays (Zigmond, Foxman, and Segall 2001; Pujic et al. 2009). Boyden chambers consist of a porous membrane separating two compartments within a tissue culture vessel (Boyden 1962) (Figure 11.1a). Cells are placed in the top compartment and a chemoattractant is placed in the lower compartment. The chemoattractant diffuses upward, causing cells to migrate through the pores in the membrane. After a specified period of time, the number of cells in the lower and upper compartments is counted to determine the percentage of migratory cells.

The Zigmond chamber was developed to facilitate observation of the cells during migration (Zigmond 1977). A Zigmond chamber consists of a slide with two closely spaced rectangular reservoirs connected by a bridge (Figure 11.1b). A concentration gradient is established along the length of the bridge by filling one reservoir with media and the other with a chemoattractant. A population of cells attached to a coverslip is affixed to the chamber and visualized as the cells migrate toward the chemoattractant.

A third migration assay, the under-agarose assay, allows additional flexibility in the positioning of the reservoirs containing the chemoattractant (Nelson, Quie, and Simmons 1975) (Figure 11.1c). Agarose is poured into the bottom of a dish and allowed to cool and then small wells are punched out of the agarose gel. Cells and media with or without a chemoattractant are added to the wells. The chemoattractant

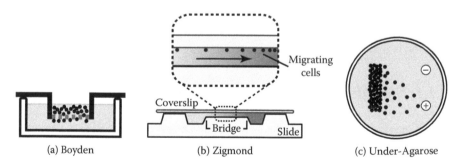

(a) Boyden   (b) Zigmond   (c) Under-Agarose

Figure 11.1
A schematic of popular cell migration assays. (a) In the Boyden assay, the percentage of cells that migrate through a porous membrane toward a chemoattractant is measured. (b) In the Zigmond assay, cells attached to a coverslip are placed in a chemoattractant gradient and their migration toward the chemoattractant is visualized using a microscope. (c) In the under-agarose assay, cells are seeded into a well cut in an agarose layer and migrate preferentially toward another well containing a chemoattractant, indicated by a "+" in the schematic. The arrangement of cells and chemoattractants in the assay is flexible since wells can be cut anywhere within the agarose.

diffuses through the agarose, causing cells to migrate under the agarose toward the signal. As with the Zigmond chambers, this process can be visualized using a microscope. By modifying the underlying substrate, the under-agarose assay can also be used to study the effect of nondiffusable signals on cell migration (Dee, Anderson, and Bizios 1999). This assay can be adapted to study chemokinesis by distributing a chemokine evenly throughout the agarose.

The under-agarose assay has a few advantages over multichamber assays such as the Boyden and Zigmond chambers. It allows for a more rapid analysis and quantification, requires a smaller sample of cells, can be run using disposable equipment, and involves only two-dimensional movement of cells (Nelson et al. 1975). However, cells migrate under the chemokine rather than through it, as in the other assays, thus making the results less physiologically relevant (Pujic et al. 2009).

11.1.3 Modeling Cell Motility

Migration of a cell population can be modeled as molecular diffusion, in which molecules move by Brownian motion and the path of an individual molecule is random. Analogously, the path of a single cell migrating on a surface in the absence of a chemoattractant or in a chemoattractant of uniform concentration can be assumed to be random. In molecular diffusion, the "random walks" of many particles have the net effect of moving molecules from a region of high concentration to a region of low concentration. Analogously, the "random walks" of many cells will result in cells moving from a region of high cell density to a region of low cell density. While molecular diffusion can be used to model cell migration, it is important to recognize that migrating cells are moving via active processes and are not actually diffusing.

Molecular diffusion is described mathematically by Fick's laws. For diffusion in one dimension, Fick's first law states that flux (J), the rate of net movement of particles across a plane perpendicular to the direction of diffusion, is proportional to the concentration gradient of the particles (Figure 11.2a):

$$J \propto \frac{dC}{dx} \tag{11.1}$$

The constant of proportionality for this relationship is the diffusion coefficient, D, which quantifies the speed of diffusion:

$$J = -D\frac{dC}{dx} \tag{11.2}$$

The units for J, D, C, and x are [mol/m²s], [m²/s], [mol/m³] and [m], respectively. The negative sign indicates that net movement is from a region of high concentration to a region of low concentration. An expression analogous to Fick's first law can be

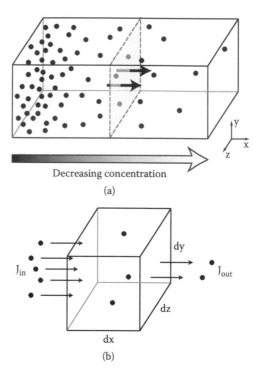

Figure 11.2

(a) Particles diffuse from a region of high concentration to a region of low concentration. The net flux (J) of particles across a plane perpendicular to the direction of diffusion is proportional to the concentration gradient of the particles. (b) The rate of change in the quantity of particles within a control volume ($dx \cdot dy \cdot dz$) is equal to the number of particles entering the control volume per unit time ($J_{in} \cdot$ area) minus the number of particles leaving the control volume per unit time ($J_{out} \cdot$ area). These relationships form the basis of Fick's laws of diffusion.

used to describe cell migration in one dimension by replacing the diffusion coefficient with the random motility coefficient (μ):

$$J = -\mu \frac{dC}{dx} \tag{11.3}$$

The random motility coefficient quantifies the speed of cell migration in the absence of a chemoattractant or when the concentration of the chemoattractant is uniform, such as in chemokinesis. The random motility coefficient has been measured for multiple cell types under different experimental conditions and is typically on the order of 10^{-8} to 10^{-7} cm²/s (Palsson and Bhatia 2004). In this experiment, you will measure the random motility coefficient of fibroblasts in the presence and absence of a chemoattractant.

Fick's second law describes how concentration changes over time as a result of diffusion (Figure 11.2b). The quantity of particles, measured in moles, within a control volume $(dx \cdot dy \cdot dz)$, is equal to the concentration of particles (C) multiplied by the volume:

$$C(dx \cdot dy \cdot dz)$$

The rate of change in the number of particles in the control volume is therefore

$$\frac{dC(dx \cdot dy \cdot dz)}{dt}$$

The rate of change in the quantity of particles in the control volume can also be written as the number of particles entering the control volume per unit time minus the number of particles leaving the control volume per unit time:

$$J_{in}(dy \cdot dz) - J_{out}(dy \cdot dz)$$

Setting these two expressions to be equal gives

$$\frac{dC(dx \cdot dy \cdot dz)}{dt} = (J_{in} - J_{out})(dy \cdot dz) \tag{11.4}$$

$$\frac{dC}{dt}dx = -dJ \tag{11.5}$$

$$\frac{dC}{dt} = -\frac{dJ}{dx} \tag{11.6}$$

Substituting Equation 11.2 into Equation 11.6 gives Fick's second law of diffusion:

$$\frac{dC}{dt} = -\frac{d}{dx}\left(-D\frac{dC}{dx}\right) \tag{11.7}$$

$$\frac{dC}{dt} = D\frac{d^2C}{dx^2} \tag{11.8}$$

Fick's second law can be used to model cell migration by again replacing the diffusion coefficient with the random motility coefficient (μ):

$$\frac{dC}{dt} = \mu \frac{d^2 C}{dx^2}$$ (11.9)

11.1.4 Measuring Cell Motility

The under-agarose assay can be used to experimentally measure the random motility coefficient for a population of cells under specific conditions (Lauffenburger, Rothman, and Zigmond 1983). Briefly, a rectangular well is cut into a layer of agarose and a cell suspension is seeded into the well. After a period of time in culture, the density of cells at different distances from the well is measured (Figure 11.3a). The density data are then fit to the solution of Equation 11.9 using the appropriate boundary conditions (Figure 11.3b). Finally, the random motility coefficient is extrapolated from the data fit. The appropriate boundary conditions are (Lauffenburger et al. 1983)

$$
\begin{aligned}
x = 0 \quad & C = C_0 \quad t > 0 \\
x \to \infty \quad & C \to 0 \quad t > 0 \\
t = 0 \quad & C = 0 \quad x > 0
\end{aligned}
$$

The first boundary condition assumes that there is a constant concentration of cells (C_0) at the well wall ($x = 0$). The second assumes that the size of the assay is larger than the distance a cell can travel during the time of the experiment. The third boundary condition assumes that there are no cells present outside the well initially. Solving Equation 11.9 with these boundary conditions gives (Lauffenburger et al. 1983)

$$C = C_0 \left[1 - erf \left\{ \frac{x}{2\sqrt{\mu t}} \right\} \right]$$ (11.10)

11.1.5 Platelet-Derived Growth Factor (PDGF)

This experiment investigates the effect of PDGF on 3T3 fibroblast migration and the corresponding motility coefficient. PDGF was one of the first growth factors to be identified and, as with many growth factors, the effects of PDGF are not limited to stimulating cell proliferation (Alberts et al. 2007). In particular, PDGF has been shown to increase fibroblast migration (Seppa et al. 1982). In the body, PDGF is important in the wound-healing response. Platelets at the site of injury release PDGF to recruit fibroblasts to the wound site and to stimulate their proliferation. To isolate the effects of PDGF on migration in this experiment, cell proliferation will be inhibited by pretreating the cells with mitomycin C, which cross-links DNA and prevents replication. It is frequently used to prevent proliferation of feeder cells that support the maintenance of embryonic stem cells in culture.

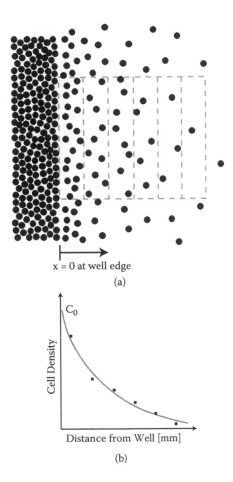

$x = 0$ at well edge

(a)

(b)

Figure 11.3
(a) To measure the motility coefficient using an under-agarose assay, a rectangular well is cut into a layer of agarose and a cell suspension is seeded into the well. After time in culture, the density of cells at different distances from the well edge is determined. Cell density is found by dividing the number of cells within defined regions (shown as row of boxes) by the area of that region. Distance is measured from the well edge to the midpoint of each region. For clarity, only migration of cells from the right side of the well is shown in the schematic. (b) The density data, obtained experimentally, are fit to the diffusion model of cell migration and the random motility coefficient is extrapolated from the data fit.

11.2 Learning Objectives

The objectives of this experiment are to

- Learn to perform an under-agarose assay
- Fit experimental data to a mathematical model to extract the motility coefficient of 3T3 fibroblasts
- Quantify the effect of PDGF on 3T3 fibroblast migration

11.3 Overview of Experiment

The overall procedure for this experiment involves preparing an under-agarose assay and observing the migration of 3T3 fibroblasts in the presence or absence of PDGF. Micrographs of cells that have migrated from their original position will be captured and analyzed. The results from the assay will be fit to a model of cell migration and used to calculate the motility coefficient of 3T3 fibroblasts in the presence or absence of PDGF.

11.4 Safety Notes

Use good lab practices and review all relevant MSDSs.

11.5 Materials

In addition to the general equipment and supplies, the following are needed to complete this experiment:

11.5.1 Reagents and Consumables

- ~1×10^6 3T3 Cells in monolayer culture (e.g., 1×100 mm confluent dish). Instructors will pretreat the cell cultures with 10 µg/mL mitomycin C for 3 h prior to the lab to prevent proliferation during the course of the experiment.
- Agarose
- DMEM (high glucose)
- Bovine calf serum (BCS)
- 2X Hank's balanced salt solution (HBSS)
- Penicillin/streptomycin (P/S)
- 0.25% Trypsin with EDTA (1X)
- Trypan blue
- 50 µg/mL Platelet-derived growth factor (PDGF)
- Sterile plastic spatula

11.5.2 Equipment and Supplies

- Hot plate
- Thermometer

11.6 Recipes

2X HBSS. Dilute 10X HBSS fivefold in dH_2O.

4 mM HCl in 0.1% BSA. Add 40 µL of 1 M HCl and 10 mg bovine serum albumin (BSA) to 10 mL dH_2O. Mix well and filter through a 0.2 µm syringe filter into a sterile container.

50 µg/mL PDGF stock. Reconstitute lyophilized PDGF, as supplied, to 50 µg/mL in sterile 4 mM HCl in 0.1% BSA. Prepare 20 µL aliquots and store at –20°C or –80°C. Avoid repeated freeze–thaw cycles.

11.7 Methods

11.7.1 Session 1: Prepare the Agarose Plates

1. In a 37°C water bath, warm ~10 mL BCS, ~1 mL of P/S, and ~35 mL of DMEM.

2. Preheat a second water bath to 70°C.

3. Fill a 500 mL beaker approximately halfway with water and bring it to a boil on a hot plate.

4. Prepare the agarose solution:

   a. Weigh out 0.48 g of agarose in 50 mL conical tube.

   b. Add 10 mL dH_2O to the conical tube.

   c. Place the tube in the boiling water with the lid loosely attached.

   d. Allow the agarose to dissolve fully. The solution's appearance will change from cloudy to clear once the agarose has dissolved.

5. Prepare the biosafety cabinet (BSC) for use by wiping it down with 70% ethanol and arranging necessary reagents and disposables.

6. Prepare heat-inactivated media:

   a. In the BSC, combine 31.6 mL DMEM, 8 mL BCS, and 0.4 mL P/S in a sterile conical tube.

   b. Split the media equally into two 50 mL conical tubes. To one tube, add 10 mL of 2X HBSS.

   c. Cap both tubes and warm their contents to 70°C in a water bath.

7. Label an empty 15 mL conical tube "+PDGF" and another "excess agarose." Place a thermometer in the tube labeled "excess agarose." The thermometer does not need to be sterile, just lightly sprayed with ethanol, because the excess agarose will not be used in culture. Set both tubes aside in the BSC. Label three wells each of a six-well plate "–PDGF" and "+PDGF." You will need these items nearby later in the protocol.

8. Cast the agarose gels in the six-well plate after the agarose has fully dissolved (see Step 4) *and* the medium has reached 70°C (see Step 6):

   a. Within the BSC, transfer the media/HBSS mixture to the tube containing the agarose.

   b. Mix well with a pipette, being careful not to create air bubbles.

c. Transfer 10 mL of the agarose/media/HBSS solution to the "+PDGF" tube and then 10 mL to the "excess agarose" tube.

d. Use the remaining agarose/media/HBSS solution to cast the agarose gels that do not contain PDGF. To do this, add 3 mL of the agarose/media/HBSS solution to each of the three wells labeled "–PDGF" in the six-well plate.

e. Monitor the temperature of the agarose/media/HBSS in the 15 mL conical tubes. Once the temperature reaches 40°C, add 20 μL of the 50 μg/mL PDGF stock to the "+PDGF" tube.

f. Mix well with a pipette, being careful not to create air bubbles.

g. Add 3 mL of this solution to each of the three wells labeled "+PDGF" in the six-well plate.

h. Swirl the plate gently if the agarose does not cover the entire well surface.

i. Remove any bubbles by aspirating with a Pasteur pipette.

j. Set the plate aside in the BSC and allow the agarose to solidify, ~15 min.

9. Store the agarose gels and the tube of heat-deactivated media in the refrigerator until the next session.

11.7.2 Session 2: Seed the Cells to Initiate the Migration Assay

1. In a 37°C water bath, warm ~4 mL of trypsin and ~20 mL of heat-deactivated media (prepared in session 1).

2. Place the agarose gels in the incubator to equilibrate with the environment.

3. Prepare the BSC for use by wiping it down with 70% ethanol and arranging necessary reagents and disposables.

4. Prepare the 3T3 cells for seeding:

a. Remove 3T3 cells from incubator.

b. View the cells under the microscope. Note the cell morphology and extent of confluence.

c. In the BSC, trypsinize the cells (refer to trypsinization protocol in Appendix 1) and rinse once in 10 mL of heat-deactivated media.

d. Remove a small sample of the cell suspension and count the cells using a hemacytometer (refer to hemacytometer protocol in Appendix 2).

e. Spin down the cell suspension and resuspend the cells to achieve a final concentration of 2×10^6 cells/mL. You will need at least 0.15 mL of the cell suspension at this concentration.

5. Create wells for cell seeding within the gels:

a. Remove the six-well plate from incubator and transfer it to the BSC.

b. In the center of each well, make two parallel cuts in the agarose by pressing a sterile plastic spatula straight down through the agarose. The distance between the cuts should be slightly larger than the diameter of the Pasteur pipette (~1–1.5 mm). Do not scratch the surface of the wells by dragging the spatula along it.

   c. Remove the agarose between the two cuts by aspiration through a Pasteur pipette. If possible, aspirate the agarose without allowing the pipette tip to touch the well surface to prevent scratching the well surface.

6. Seed the cells into the agarose gel:

   a. Mix the cell suspension thoroughly.

   b. Fill each well with 25 μL of the cell suspension.

7. Transfer the six-well plate and any remaining cell suspension into the incubator.

8. After 10 min, check for any cell leakage under the agarose using a microscope. If there is significant cell leakage, cut a new well ~1 cm from the previous well and seed with cells as before. If there is no leakage, capture at least one digital image using a 20X objective near the center of a well.

9. Transfer the assay to the incubator for 24–48 h.

11.7.3 Session 3: Document Cell Motility

1. Remove the six-well plate from the incubator.

2. Add three to four drops of media or PBS to the gels. This will improve the quality of the image.

3. Using transmitted light, visualize the cells under the microscope, noting differences in the distance cells migrated in each well.

4. Capture at least one representative digital image using a 20X objective near the center of each well. Find a location where the well edge is straight and the cells have not pulled away from the well edge. The images should contain the well edge and the cell that migrated the farthest from the edge. If not, capture multiple, overlapping frames. *Note: these images are critical for data analysis, so they must be in focus and of the correct region.*

5. Obtain a calibration image so that you will be able to determine the distance the cells have migrated. You may get a calibration image from your instructor or acquire an image of a stage micrometer or hemacytometer grid using the same magnification as in the micrographs.

11.8 Data Processing and Reporting

Briefly report the results of your experiment in paragraph and graphical form. Each of the key results to report in text, figure, and/or table format is described next.

1. In one professional-quality figure with multiple panels, include the micrograph captured immediately after cell seeding ($t = 0$) and one representative micrograph per experimental condition showing the well edge and most distant cell. Include a scale bar.

2. Determine the cell density as a function of distance for each experimental condition:

TABLE 11.1

Suggested Format for Presenting Cell Migration Data

Distance (x; mm)	Cell Density (C; cells/mm²)							
	−PDGF				+PDGF			
	Well 1	Well 2	Well 3	Mean	Well 1	Well 2	Well 3	Mean
0.05								
0.15								
0.25								
0.35								
...								

a. Superimpose a grid of known size (e.g., 0.1 × 0.5 mm) on each image, as shown in Figure 11.3a.

b. Count the number of cells, or nuclei, within each grid for one row of the image. *Note: Cells straddling the borders can be placed in either the left or right grid as long as this is done consistently.*

c. Divide the cell counts by the area of each grid to calculate cell density.

d. Organize your data in a table similar to Table 11.1, using the midpoint of each grid as the distance from the well.

3. Use the mean cell density values to calculate the motility coefficient (μ) for each experimental condition. Specifically, rearrange Equation 11.10 as shown:

$$C = C_0 \left[1 - erf \left\{ \frac{x}{2\sqrt{\mu t}} \right\} \right] \qquad \text{(11.10 repeated)}$$

$$2\sqrt{t} \, erf^{-1} \left(1 - \frac{C}{C_0} \right) = \frac{1}{\sqrt{\mu}} x \qquad \text{(11.11)}$$

A linear regression of the left side of Equation 11.11 versus distance from the well (x) yields a slope equal to $1/\sqrt{\mu}$. It is not possible to evaluate the left side of Equation 11.11, however, because the density of cells at the well edge (C_0) is unknown. C_0 is the same for both experimental conditions. There are two approaches to determine C_0:

Method 1: use a software package to perform a least squares regression to determine both unknown parameters, μ and C_0, simultaneously.

Method 2: use an estimate for C_0. The estimate can be made from the data you collect, trial and error to optimize the regression (similar to method 1), or in some other way clearly explained in your report. If you estimate C_0, perform a sensitivity analysis to determine how the estimate affects the motility coefficient and the conclusions drawn.

4. Generate one graph showing the mean experimental data for each condition (x-axis: distance from well edge; y-axis: cell density). Superimpose on the experimental data

the predictions of the migration growth model using the calculated motility coefficient. Discuss how well the model fits the experimental data and suggest possible reasons for discrepancies.

5. Briefly describe the effect that PDGF had on the motility of the cell populations.

11.9 Prelab Questions

1. Calculate the concentration of PDGF in the agarose during the migration assay.

2. When would it be necessary for a tissue-engineered medical product to induce a high cell motility coefficient? Provide one or more examples.

3. Why is it important to allow the agarose solution to cool to 40°C before adding PDGF?

4. Why is it necessary to seed such a high concentration of cells in each well?

11.10 Postlab Questions

1. Explain why it would be difficult to interpret the experimental results if the cells were allowed to proliferate during the experiment.

2. Describe an alternate method that could be used to increase the motility of 3T3 cells in the under-agarose assay.

3. Briefly describe how you would determine, statistically, if the motility coefficient for the cells with and without PDGF is significantly different.

4. Compare your calculated or estimated value of C_0 to the values found from a similar experiment by Lauffenburger and colleagues (1983). Are the values similar? Why or why not?

5. Compare your calculated values of μ to a value or values reported in the literature for any cell type under any experimental conditions. Are the values the same order of magnitude? Discuss similarities and differences in the experiment and how these may be reflected in order of magnitude of the motility coefficient. Cite your source(s).

6. If you were to repeat the experiment again, what modifications would you make?

References

Boyden, S. 1962. The chemotactic effect of mixtures of antibody and antigen on polymorphonuclear leucocytes. *Journal of Experimental Medicine* 115:453–466.

Dee, K. C., T. T. Anderson, and R. Bizios. 1999. Osteoblast population migration characteristics on substrates modified with immobilized adhesive peptides. *Biomaterials* 20 (3): 221–227.

Lauffenburger, D., C. Rothman, and S. H. Zigmond. 1983. Measurement of leukocyte motility and chemotaxis parameters with a linear under-agarose migration assay. *Journal of Immunology* 131 (2): 940–947.

Nelson, R. D., P. G. Quie, and R. L. Simmons. 1975. Chemotaxis under agarose: A new and simple method for measuring chemotaxis and spontaneous migration of human polymorphonuclear leukocytes and monocytes. *Journal of Immunology* 115 (6): 1650–1656.

Palsson, B. O., and S. N. Bhatia. 2004. *Tissue engineering.* Upper Saddle River, NJ: Pearson Education.

Pujic, Z., D. Mortimer, J. Feldner, and G. J. Goodhill. 2009. Assays for eukaryotic cell chemotaxis. *Combinatorial Chemistry & High Throughput Screening* 12 (6): 580–588.

Seppa, H., G. Grotendorst, S. Seppa, E. Schiffmann, and G. R. Martin. 1982. Platelet-derived growth factor in chemotactic for fibroblasts. *Journal of Cell Biology* 92 (2): 584–588.

Zigmond, S. H. 1977. Ability of polymorphonuclear leukocytes to orient in gradients of chemotactic factors. *Journal of Cell Biology* 75 (2 Pt 1): 606–616.

Zigmond, S. H., E. F. Foxman, and J. E. Segall. 2001. Chemotaxis assays for eukaryotic cells. In *Current protocols in cell biology.* New York: John Wiley & Sons, Inc.

Characterizing Matrix Remodeling through Collagen Gel Contraction

12.1 Background

The extracellular matrix (ECM) is an interconnected network of macromolecules including collagens, laminins, fibronectin, proteoglycans, and glycosaminoglycans. Cells synthesize, secrete, degrade, and reorganize their surrounding ECM during development, growth, wound healing, and normal tissue maintenance. ECM remodeling also occurs in pathogenic processes such as fibrosis, tumor formation, and metastasis.

Tissue engineers apply fundamental knowledge of matrix remodeling to guide cells through the similar processes needed to develop an engineered tissue *in vitro*. Furthermore, it may be important for tissue engineers to control wound healing and subsequent remodeling after implantation of a tissue-engineered medical product (TEMP) in order to achieve long-term clinical success. Experimental models of cells embedded within a three-dimensional ECM are frequently used to study the process of matrix remodeling (Bell, Ivarsson, and Merrill 1979). The most common models involve fibroblasts embedded within a hydrated collagen network or gel.

Three experimental models of fibroblast–collagen gel remodeling have been widely used: free floating, constrained, and stress–relaxed (Grinnell and Petroll 2010) (Figure 12.1). In all three models, a mixture of fibroblasts and collagen is cast into a culture dish and allowed to polymerize. With time in culture, the fibroblasts attempt to reorganize the randomly oriented collagen fibrils. In free-floating experiments, the gels are released from the culture dish shortly after polymerization. As a result, the gels contract as cells remodel the matrix. The degree of organization of collagen matrix is quantified by the measured reduction in diameter of the construct over time. In the constrained model, the polymerized gels remain attached to the

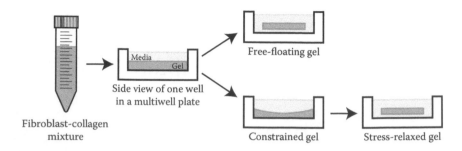

Figure 12.1

In the three common experiments used to study fibroblast–collagen gel remodeling, a mixture of fibroblasts and collagen is polymerized within wells of a culture plate. In free-floating experiments, the resulting gels are released from the well shortly after polymerization and contract as cells remodel the collagen matrix. In the constrained model, the polymerized gels remain attached to the well throughout the experiment so that changes in gel geometry are restricted to changes in thickness. A stress–relaxation experiment involves releasing gels that have been cultured in a constrained configuration and allowing them to contract upon their release.

culture vessel throughout the experiment and changes in gel geometry are restricted to changes in thickness. A stress–relaxation experiment involves releasing gels that have been cultured in a constrained configuration and allowing them to contract upon their release.

The mechanism by which gel contraction occurs and the morphology of the fibroblasts depend on the experimental model used (Grinnell and Petroll 2010). Specifically, free-floating gels contract when indwelling cells develop a highly branched morphology and exert rearward force on their local collagen network (Grinnell and Petroll 2010). In constrained matrices, the collagen network resists the forces exerted by the cells, leading to tension within the matrix and cells with a bipolar morphology (Grinnell and Petroll 2010). When constrained gels are released, such as in a stress–relaxation experiment, the cells shorten in length, causing overall gel contraction (Grinnell and Petroll 2010).

Cell morphology can be quantified using a dimensionless parameter called the shape index (SI):

$$SI = \frac{4\pi A}{P^2}$$

where A is the projected cell area and P is the cell perimeter. The shape index ranges from 1 for a perfect circle to 0 for a straight line. A spherical cell has a large shape index, a bipolar cell has an intermediate shape index, and a highly branched cell has a small shape index.

In addition to serving as a useful model for studying matrix remodeling, fibroblast–collagen gels can be used as tissue substitutes. One of the first TEMPs contains a fibroblast–collagen gel similar to the experimental models under investigation here. Apligraf® consists of allogeneic neonatal fibroblasts grown in a collagen gel with an overlay of allogeneic neonatal keratinocytes (Wilkins et al. 1994). The bilayer structure of Apligraf resembles the dermis and epidermis of native skin. Apligraf contributes to the healing of chronic foot or leg ulcers by delivering growth factors and cells to the site of injury.

Produced by Organogenesis, Apligraf was approved by the FDA in 1997 and initially experienced a long period of stagnant sales but has since demonstrated potential for continued commercial success (Lysaght, Jaklenec, and Deweerd 2008). Other tissue-engineered skin products use a similar approach of embedding viable cells within a three-dimensional, hydrated matrix that is biological, synthetic, or a combination of both (Shevchenko, James, and James 2010).

12.2 Learning Objectives

The objectives of this experiment are to

- Investigate the interaction between cells and the ECM using a fibroblast–collagen gel *in vitro* culture model
- Using statistics, determine whether the extent of matrix remodeling depends on the density of cells within the gel
- Measure and compare the shape index of cells within free-floating and constrained gels

12.3 Overview of Experiment

The overall procedure for this experiment involves seeding a mixture of fibroblasts and collagen in multiwell culture plates using proper sterile techniques, letting the mixtures polymerize, detaching the gels from the wells, and measuring the diameter of the gels after the fibroblasts remodel the collagen matrix (Figure 12.2). Two gels will not be detached from the culture well and instead will be used to compare the morphology of cells within free-floating and constrained gels. The experiment will be performed for different fibroblast concentrations (0, 0.1×10^6, 0.2×10^6, and 0.4×10^6 cells/mL) with a collagen concentration of 1.5 mg/mL for all samples.

12.4 Safety Notes

Use good lab practices and review all relevant MSDSs.

12.5 Materials

In addition to the general equipment and supplies, the following are needed to complete this experiment:

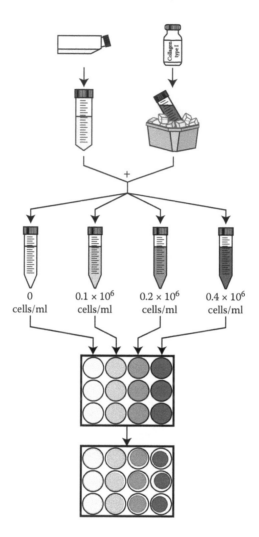

Figure 12.2
Schematic of the collagen gel contraction experiment that will be performed in this lab. Fibroblasts are released from monolayer culture with trypsin and mixed, at various densities, with collagen. The fibroblast–collagen mixtures are polymerized in multiwell plates and, with time in culture, the fibroblasts remodel the collagen networks in which they are embedded. This remodeling results in visible changes in gel diameter.

12.5.1 Reagents and Consumables

- $>5 \times 10^6$ 3T3 Cells in monolayer culture (e.g., 2×100 mm confluent dishes)
- 3T3 Media (recipe follows)
- 3X DMEM
- 3 mg/mL Type I rat tail tendon collagen in 0.02 N acetic acid (must form gel; e.g., from BD Biosciences)

- 0.25% Trypsin with EDTA (1X)
- Trypan blue
- 1X Phosphate-buffered saline (PBS)
- 4 mM Calcein AM in DMSO (EX: 494 nm, EM: 517 nm)
- Sterile spatula

12.5.2 Equipment and Supplies

- Ruler
- Ice bucket or cooler with ice
- Microscope equipped for fluorescence (EX: 494 nm, EM: 517 nm) and digital imaging

12.6 Recipes

3T3 Media. Add 50 mL bovine calf serum (BCS) and 5 mL of 100X penicillin/streptomycin (P/S) to 445 mL of high glucose DMEM.

3X DMEM. Dilute powdered DMEM in a third of the recommended volume of deionized H$_2$O (dH$_2$O), add 11.1 mg/mL NaHCO$_3$, stir well, adjust pH to 7.4, and filter through a 0.2 μm syringe filter into a sterile container. Make 5 mL aliquots and store at –20°C.

Collagen. Dilute the collagen as supplied to a final concentration of 3 mg/mL with 0.02 N sterile acetic acid.

1X PBS. Add 50 mL 10X PBS (with Ca^{2+} and Mg^{2+}) to 400 mL dH$_2$O. Mix well, adjust pH to 7.4 with HCl and NaOH, bring total volume to 500 mL with dH$_2$O, and either sterile-filter through a 0.2 μm filter or autoclave.

12.7 Methods

12.7.1 Session 1: Prepare Cell-Seeded Collagen Gels

1. In a 37°C water bath, warm 3T3 media, a 5 mL aliquot of 3X DMEM, and ~8 mL of trypsin.
2. Prepare the biosafety cabinet (BSC) for use by wiping it down with 70% ethanol and arranging necessary reagents and disposables.
3. In the BSC, dilute the 3 mg/mL collagen stock solution with 3X DMEM to make 12 mL of 2 mg/mL collagen in DMEM. Cap the conical tube and place the solution in an ice bath until needed.
4. Prepare 3T3 cells for seeding:
   a. Remove 3T3 cells from the incubator.

TABLE 12.1

Recipes for Preparation of Collagen Gels with Varying Cell Density

Tube No.	Vol. Cell Suspension (mL)	Vol. Collagen Solution (mL)	Vol. 3T3 Media (mL)	Final Cell Concentration (cells/mL)	Final Collagen Concentration (mg/mL)
1	0.8	2.4	0	0.4×10^6	1.5
2	0.4	2.4	0.4	0.2×10^6	1.5
3	0.3	3.6	0.9	0.1×10^6	1.5
4	0	2.4	0.8	0	1.5

    b. View the cells under microscope. Note the extent of confluence in your lab notebook.

    c. Trypsinize the cells (refer to trypsinization protocol in Appendix 1).

    d. Spin the cell suspension down in a centrifuge at 300 g, discard the supernatant, and resuspend the pellet in 2 mL of 3T3 media.

    e. Count the cells using a hemacytometer (refer to hemacytometer protocol in Appendix 2).

    f. Dilute the suspension to a final concentration of 1.6×10^6 cells/mL.

5. In 15 mL conical tubes, mix the collagen solution, cell suspension, and 3T3 media according to the recipes in Table 12.1. Notice that the final volume in tube 3 should be larger since this is the solution from which the constrained gels will be made. Mix the solutions well but avoid making bubbles.

6. Pipette 0.8 mL of the cell–collagen mixtures into each well of a 12-well plate, as shown in Figure 12.2. All samples are prepared in triplicate.

7. In a second 12-well plate, prepare two additional gels with 0.1×10^6 cells/mL to be cultured in the constrained configuration (i.e., attached to the culture dish).

8. Allow the mixtures to gel in the incubator for 15 min.

9. After the gels have polymerized, detach the collagen constructs from the sides and bottoms of the culture wells. *Note: This step does not apply to the two constructs that will be cultured in the constrained configuration.*

    a. In the BSC, detach the collagen gels by carefully tracing the perimeters of each with a sterile spatula.

    b. Holding the plate at a slight angle, use the spatula to detach the gel from the bottom of the well by sliding the top of the gel toward the center of the well. Rotate the plate and repeat until each gel appears to be free floating.

    c. Gently tilt or swirl the plate to verify that the gels are completely detached from wells.

10. Add 0.5 mL of 3T3 media to each gel, including the constrained gels, and return plates to the incubator. Culture the constructs at least overnight and up to a week before measuring gel contraction (session 2). For extended cultures, media should be changed every 2–3 days and the constrained gels may detach from the well; therefore, cultures of a few days are recommended.

12.7.2 Session 2: Measure Gel Contraction and Cell Morphology

1. Measure the diameter of each construct:

   a. Remove the 12-well plate containing the free-floating constructs from the incubator.

   b. Place the plate directly on top of a ruler. Measure and record the diameter of each construct in two perpendicular directions. The average of these two measurements should be taken as the estimate of construct diameter. Alternatively, use a digital camera or camera phone to take a digital image with the plate and ruler in the same frame and use ImageJ (or a similar program) to determine construct diameter or area.

2. Compare cell morphology in a free-floating and constrained construct:

   a. Thaw calcein AM and dilute 2 μL in 4 mL of PBS. Calcein AM is a membrane-permeable molecule that is enzymatically cleaved within the cytoplasm of viable cells to produce an intensely fluorescent dye, calcein (EX: 494 nm, EM: 517 nm).

   b. Replace the media in the constrained constructs and two of the free-floating, 0.1×10^6 cells/mL constructs with 1 mL of the calcein AM-PBS solution.

   c. Incubate the constructs at 37°C in calcein AM for 10 min.

   d. Set up the microscope for fluorescence imaging; use a filter cube compatible with calcein AM. Allow the lamp to warm up ~15 min.

   e. View labeled cells within the constructs using fluorescence microscopy and a high-powered objective. *Note: Exposure of the samples to the fluorescent lamp should be minimized to avoid photobleaching, which is the destruction of the dye and results in diminished brightness. If the constructs move around too much, remove most of the fluid so that they settle to the dish surface.*

   f. Capture digital pictures of five representative cells in both the free-floating and constrained constructs. Save the images for later image analysis.

3. Obtain a calibration image so that you will be able to add a scale bar to representative micrographs when documenting your results. You may get a calibration image from your instructor or acquire an image of a stage micrometer or hemacytometer grid using the same magnification as in the micrographs.

12.8 Data Processing and Reporting

Briefly report the results of your experiment in paragraph and graphical form. Each of the key results to report in text, figure, and/or table format is described next.

1. Include a bar graph displaying the average gel diameter for each of the experimental conditions. Include and label error bars. Indicate the number of observations represented by each data point.

2. Statistical analysis: perform a one-way ANOVA on the preceding data to determine the effect of cell density on extent of gel contraction. Report the degrees of freedom, critical F-value corresponding to $p < 0.05$, the p-value obtained from your data, and the statistical power. Use an appropriate post hoc test as needed to test for pairwise differences.

3. Include representative images of cells within the free-floating and constrained gels. Using image processing software, measure the area and perimeter of the five representative cells in both the free-floating and constrained constructs. Calculate and report the shape index as mean ± standard deviation.

12.9 Prelab Questions

1. Calculate the volume of 3 mg/mL collagen stock solution and the volume of 3X DMEM that will be used to make 12 mL of 2 mg/mL collagen in DMEM as described in session 1, step 3.

2. Why is it necessary to store the diluted collagen solution on ice after it is diluted in media but not before?

3. What do you expect the relationship to be between initial cell concentration and collagen gel contraction? Briefly explain.

4. Compare the concentration of serum in standard fibroblast media to the concentration within the wells after the addition of 0.5 mL of media at the end of day 1 (estimate serum concentration as a percentage of total volume). If they are different, what might be the effect on the cells and why?

5. Recently, a modification to the classic gel contraction assay was proposed by Ilagan et al. (2010). Instead of casting disc-shaped gels within a multiwell plate (Figure 12.3a), the new assay casts long, thin, cable-like gels within capillary tubes (Figure 12.3b). The authors state that the classic method results in inaccuracies by attempting to quantify volumetric changes by measuring one-dimensional changes in gel diameter. They propose that the new method more accurately quantifies contractility "by reducing

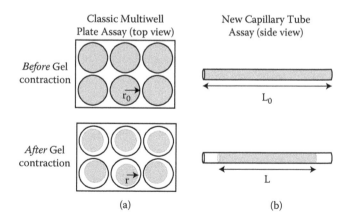

Figure 12.3
Schematics of the (a) classic gel contraction assay in a multiwell plate and (b) new gel contraction assay in capillary tubes.

the collagen gel dimensions to a single, linear measurement." In reality, both assays attempt to characterize three-dimensional contraction of a cylinder by measuring a decrease in one dimension; the classic assay tracks cylinder diameter (or radius) while the new assay tracks cylinder height. Both assays neglect any changes in the perpendicular direction.

a. Assume that the gels in both assays contract uniformly resulting in a 10% decrease in both gel radius and height. Calculate the volume of these contracted gels as a fraction of their initial volume. Calculate the volume of the contracted gels that would be estimated from the classic assay (neglecting changes in height) and the new assay (neglecting changes in radius). Calculate the percentage error in the measurement for each assay. Which assay is more accurate? Why? Is the trend the same when the gel contracts more than 10%?

b. The calculation in part (5a) assumes complete precision in the gel geometry measurements. Taking into account how the contraction data are collected in the lab, what advantage does the new assay offer?

c. Based on the preceding assumptions and calculations, which assay is more accurate? Which assay is more precise? Briefly explain your answer.

12.10 Postlab Questions

1. Estimate (order of magnitude) the collagen composition, as percentage wet weight, in the contracted gels and compare this estimate to a typical collagen composition for mature human connective tissues. Cite your source(s) of information for native collagen composition. How might differences in collagen composition of the native and engineered tissues affect their function?

2. The active role that cells play in the remodeling process can be inferred by comparing the size of the cell-seeded gels to the cell-free control gels:

   a. Briefly describe a follow-up experiment to demonstrate clearly that the decrease in gel size is a result of matrix remodeling—not matrix degradation. Explicitly state the hypothesis of your experiment.

   b. Briefly describe a future experiment to investigate the molecular mechanism by which cells actively remodel the collagen gel. Explicitly state the hypothesis of your experiment.

3. Identify and briefly explain three advantages and three disadvantages associated with using cell-seeded collagen gels as TEMPs. The advantages and disadvantages may be related to any stage of commercialization, including product development, manufacturing, distribution, and clinical implementation.

4. Compare the results of your analysis of cell morphology with previous findings summarized in a review entitled "Fibroblast Biology in Three-Dimensional Collagen Networks" (Grinnell 2003). How were your methods similar? Different? How might these differences affect the results?

References

Bell, E., B. Ivarsson, and C. Merrill. 1979. Production of a tissue-like structure by contraction of collagen lattices by human fibroblasts of different proliferative potential in vitro. *Proceedings of National Academy of Sciences USA* 76 (3): 1274–1278.

Grinnell, F. 2003. Fibroblast biology in three-dimensional collagen matrices. *Trends in Cell Biology* 13 (5): 264–269.

Grinnell, F., and W. M. Petroll. 2010. Cell motility and mechanics in three-dimensional collagen matrices. *Annual Review of Cell and Developmental Biology* 26:335–361.

Ilagan, R., K. Guthrie, S. Quinlan, H. S. Rapoport, S. Jones, A. Church, J. Basu, and J. Ludlow. 2010. Linear measurement of cell contraction in a capillary collagen gel system. *Biotechniques* 48 (2): 153–155.

Lysaght, M. J., A. Jaklenec, and E. Deweerd. 2008. Great expectations: Private sector activity in tissue engineering, regenerative medicine, and stem cell therapeutics. *Tissue Engineering Part A* 14 (2): 305–315.

Shevchenko, R. V., S. L. James, and S. E. James. 2010. A review of tissue-engineered skin bioconstructs available for skin reconstruction. *Journal of Royal Society Interface* 7 (43): 229–258.

Wilkins, L. M., S. R. Watson, S. J. Prosky, S. F. Meunier, and N. L. Parenteau. 1994. Development of a bilayered living skin construct for clinical applications. *Biotechnology and Bioengineering* 43 (8): 747–756.

Chapter **13**

Effect of Substrate Stiffness on Cell Differentiation

13.1 Background

The extracellular matrix (ECM) provides mechanical support for surrounding cells as well as biochemical and biophysical signals that influence cell behavior. The modulus of elasticity E, or "stiffness," is a material property of the ECM that anchorage-dependent cells sense and respond to by altering migration, differentiation, proliferation, and morphology (Discher, Janmey, and Wang 2005). E is the tensile stress (σ, force applied per unit area) divided by the resultant strain (ε, relative change in length). At physiologically appropriate strains, the degree of stiffness varies dramatically between tissues; brain ($E_{brain} \sim 0.1$–1 kPa) is less stiff than striated skeletal muscle ($E_{muscle} \sim 8$–17 kPa), which is less stiff than precalcified bone ($E_{precalcified\ bone} = 25$–$40$ kPa) (Engler et al. 2006; Fung 1993). Hydrated polymer networks, called hydrogels, are useful for studying the effect of substrate stiffness on anchorage-dependent cells because they can be made with a range of material properties.

Several biodegradable and nonbiodegradable polymers can be used to fabricate hydrogels on which cells can be cultured. This experiment will utilize polyacrylamide (PA) because it is easy to vary stiffness by changing the ratio of the monomer, acrylamide, and the cross-linker, bis-acrylamide (Pelham and Wang 1997). Other advantages of PA include that (1) it is transparent, allowing observation of cells growing on top or of objects suspended within the hydrogel; (2) the pore size of the hydrogel is on the order of 100 nm, which prevents cell infiltration; and (3) passive adsorption of proteins to acrylamide is minimal, which means that only adhesive molecules intentionally cross-linked to the surface can serve as ligands for cell attachment.

PA hydrogels are composed of acrylamide and bis-acrylamide monomers in a specified ratio, and the elastic modulus has been reported for many combinations of acrylamide and bis-acrylamide. Nevertheless, it is necessary to verify hydrogel stiffness under the experimental conditions used because of variability due to changes in polymerization kinetics, the number of free radicals present, the presence of salts or alcohols, and the choice of the solvent in which the reaction takes place (Tse and Engler 2010; Damljanovic, Lagerholm, and Jacobson 2005).

Three common methods to measure hydrogel stiffness are tensile testing on a macroscopic level, atomic force microscopy (AFM), and measuring microscopic hydrogel deformations under the weight of a small steel ball (Beningo, Lo, and Wang 2002). Specifically, the size and density of the ball determine the amount of stress applied to the hydrogel, the resulting strain is measured optically, and the modulus of the hydrogel is approximated. This method uses the same principles as AFM but without the need for expensive, specialized equipment.

As noted before, the "microball" method involves measuring micrometer-scale deformations that occur within the hydrogel under the weight of a steel ball. Deformations within the hydrogel can be visualized by adding fluorescent microspheres into the acrylamide mixture prior to polymerization (Figure 13.1a). The diameter of the microspheres is roughly 1/1000 that of the steel ball. Using an inverted microscope equipped for fluorescence, it is possible to focus on the microspheres located at the very top surface of the gel.

When a steel ball is dropped onto the hydrogel, the hydrogel beneath the ball compresses, and the microspheres move into a lower focal plane (Figure 13.1b). The distance (d) between the focal point of the microsphere before and after deformation is used to calculate E. In practice, it is easier to focus on a microsphere directly under the ball first, carefully remove the ball with a magnet, and then measure the

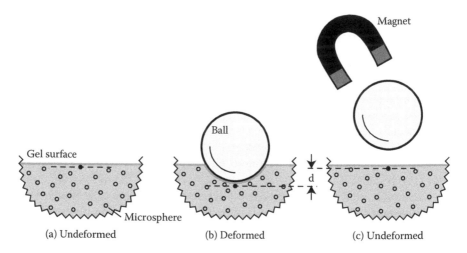

Figure 13.1
(a) PA hydrogel stiffness can be determined experimentally by embedding fluorescent microspheres within the hydrogel. (b) When a small steel ball is dropped onto the hydrogel surface, the hydrogel deforms and the microspheres displace. The position of a single microsphere directly under the ball is determined by focusing on it with a microscope. (c) The ball is removed with a magnet and the unde-formed position of the same microsphere is determined by adjusting the focal plane. The distance (d) between the deformed and undeformed focal planes is used to calculate the hydrogel stiffness.

undeformed position after the ball is removed (Figure 13.1c). The equation relating hydrogel deformation (d) to hydrogel stiffness (E) is (Damljanovic et al. 2005; Johnson 1987)

$$E = \frac{\pi\left(1-v^2\right)r^{\frac{5}{2}}g\left(\rho_b - \rho_f\right)}{d^{\frac{3}{2}}}$$

(13.1)

where
v is the Poisson ratio (approximately 0.45 for PA) (Engler et al. 2004)
r is the radius of the steel ball
g is the gravitational constant
ρ_b is the density of the ball
ρ_f is the density of the solution hydrating the hydrogel

This experiment will demonstrate that substrate stiffness affects cell function by investigating the differentiation of a preosteoblast mouse cell line, MC3T3-E1 (Khatiwala, Peyton, and Putnam 2006). Osteoblasts are the cells responsible for deposition of new bone during bone growth and remodeling. Bone ECM is primarily composed of type I collagen mineralized with calcium phosphate; thus, the deposition of calcium phosphate is a marker for the mature osteoblast phenotype (Alberts et al. 2007).

Von Kossa staining is a widely used method for detecting the presence of phosphate and, although not specific to calcium phosphate, positive von Kossa staining is commonly interpreted as evidence of bone formation (Bonewald et al. 2003). In the von Kossa method, phosphates present in the sample react with silver nitrate to produce a dark precipitate that can be visualized with a transmitted microscope. In this experiment, MC3T3-E1 will be grown on PA hydrogels of varying stiffness, and maturation of these cells toward the mature osteoblast phenotype will be qualitatively assessed using the von Kossa method. The ability to control cell differentiation is important for tissue-engineering applications—in particular, applications involving embryonic and adult stem cells.

13.2 Learning Objectives

The objectives of this experiment are to

- Fabricate PA hydrogels of varying stiffness and measure their material properties
- Learn to use creative experimental methods to circumvent the need for expensive and highly specialized instruments, when possible
- Use PA hydrogels to demonstrate how substrate stiffness can affect cell function

13.3 Overview of Experiment

This experiment will investigate the effect that substrate stiffness has on differentiation of MC3T3-E1 cells. First, PA hydrogels of varying stiffness will be fabricated from mixtures of acrylamide and bis-acrylamide. To initiate polymerization, a catalyst, tetramethylethylenediamine (TEMED), and an initiator, ammonium persulfate (APS), are added and the mixture is polymerized. Polymerizing the solution sandwiched between two glass surfaces produces hydrogels that are on the order of tens to hundreds of micrometers thick (Figure 13.2).

In this experiment, the PA is polymerized between glass microscope slides treated to increase hydrophobicity and circular glass coverslips treated to increase hydrogel attachment to its surface. After polymerization, the hydrogels remain attached to the coverslips, allowing them to be handled. Since PA resists passive protein adsorption, it is necessary to use a UV-activated cross-linker called sulfo-SANPAH to functionalize the hydrogels with collagen. Next, MC3T3-E1 cells are seeded onto the collagen-coated hydrogels. After a period of time in culture, von Kossa staining is used to detect differentiation of the MC3T3-E1 cells toward the mature osteoblast phenotype.

Hydrogel thickness and stiffness will be measured on a microscope using samples that were not seeded with cells. Gel thickness will be determined by measuring the vertical distance between the focal planes at the top and bottom surfaces of the gel. Stiffness will be determined by measuring the distance between the deformed and undeformed position of a marker within the gel upon loading, as described

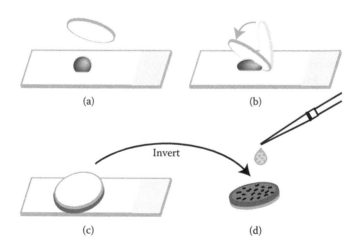

Figure 13.2
(a) To fabricate the hydrogel, a drop of acrylamide prepolymer is deposited onto a hydrophobic glass slide. (b) A round coverslip is lowered onto the drop to spread the acrylamide into a thin and uniform layer. (c) The acrylamide is allowed to polymerize in this configuration and then the coverslip, with the hydrogel attached, is removed. (d) The top surface of the hydrogel is then functionalized with collagen and seeded with cells.

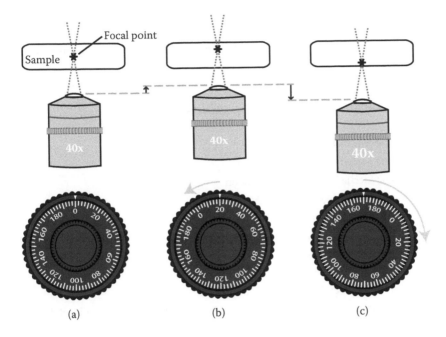

Figure 13.3
Turning the focus knob moves the microscope objective vertically and changes the height of the focal point. (a) In this schematic, the focal point is near the center of the specimen and the fine-focus knob reads "0." (b) Turning the fine-focus knob counterclockwise 20 FFUs moves the objective up and the focal point is now near the top of the specimen. (c) Turning the fine-focus knob clockwise 50 FFUs (from 20 to 170 past 0) moves the objective down and the focal point is now near the bottom of the specimen. It is possible to determine the total height of the specimen, in FFUs, by measuring the rotation required to move the focal point from the highest to lowest point within the specimen. A calibration curve to translate FFUs to microns can be generated by measuring samples of known thickness.

previously and shown in Figure 13.1. To make these measurements, it is necessary to quantify the relationship between turning the microscope's fine-focus knob and vertical movement of the focal point. In one lab session, you will generate a calibration curve to correlate rotation of the fine-focus knob, measured by the markings on the knob (or "fine-focus units," FFUs), to vertical movement of the focal point measured in microns (Figure 13.3).

13.4 Safety Notes

This protocol utilizes chemicals that are classified as serious health (APS, TEMED, formaldehyde), fire (TEMED), and physical (APS) hazards. Carefully review all relevant MSDSs and use proper personal protective equipment. Please note that TEMED is destructive to the respiratory tract and a fume hood should be used when working with it. When samples are treated with UV light, the light source should be covered with a cardboard box or similar barrier.

13.5 Materials

In addition to the general equipment and supplies, the following are needed to complete this experiment:

13.5.1 Reagents and Consumables

- 1X Phosphate-buffered saline (PBS)
- 40% (w/v) Sterile acrylamide solution
- 2% (w/v) Sterile bis-acrylamide solution
- Tetramethylethylenediamine (TEMED)
- 10% (w/v) Ammonium persulfate (APS)
- 1 mg/mL Sufosuccinimidyl-6-(4′-azido-2′-nitrophenylamino)-hexanoate (sulfo-SAN-PAH; Pierce Biotechnology)
- 50 mM HEPES buffer
- 3 mg/mL Type I collagen in 0.02 N acetic acid
- ~1 × 10^6 MC3T3-E1 cells in monolayer culture (e.g., 1 × 100 mm confluent dish)
- 0.25% Trypsin with EDTA (1X)
- Trypan blue
- MC3T3-E1 differentiation media (recipe follows)
- 4% Formaldehyde in PBS
- American MasterTech von Kossa stain kit (includes 5% silver nitrate and 5% sodium thiosulfate)
- 18 mm Circular amino-silanated coverslips (instructors will pretreat coverslips and slides within 48 h of the lab)
- 25 × 75 mm Chlorosilanated glass slides (instructors will pretreat coverslips and slides within 48 h of the lab)
- 1 μm DIA yellow-green fluorescent microspheres (EX: 505 nm, EM: 515 nm; Molecular Probes)

13.5.2 Equipment and Supplies

- Chemical fume hood
- Curved forceps (extra-fine tip)
- Alloy steel ball (1 mm DIA; McMaster-Carr)
- Slender magnet
- Vacuum desiccator (connected to vacuum line)
- UV lamp (320–365 nm) with stand and UV barrier
- Microscope with a translational stage equipped for fluorescence (EX: 505 nm, EM: 515 nm) and digital imaging

13.6 Recipes

1X PBS. Add 50 mL 10X PBS (with Ca^{2+} and Mg^{2+}) to 400 mL deionized H_2O (dH_2O). Mix well, adjust pH to 7.4 with HCl and NaOH, bring total volume to 500 mL with dH_2O, and either sterile-filter through a 0.2 μm filter or autoclave.

Acrylamide and bis-acrylamide. If supplied nonsterile, the 40% acrylamide and 2% bis-acrylamide solutions should be sterile-filtered through a 0.2 μm filter.

Fluorescent microspheres. Dilute spheres as supplied 1:10 in dH_2O prior to use.

50 mM HEPES. Dilute stock HEPES, as supplied, to 50 mM with dH_2O. Adjust pH to 8.5.

1 mg/mL Sulfo-SANPAH. Dilute sulfo-SANPAH to 1 mg/mL in dH_2O. Store this stock solution at –20°C protected from light and moisture. Dilute fivefold in 50 mM HEPES prior to use.

Type I collagen. Dilute collagen, as supplied, to 3 mg/mL in sterile 0.02 N acetic acid.

500 mM β-glycerolphosphate stock (50X). Dissolve β-glycerolphosphate disodium salt pentahydrate (MW = 306) in serum-free media at 0.15 g/mL, sterile-filter, and store at 4°C. Add to culture media 1:50 (v/v) as needed.

Ascorbic acid stock (500X). Dissolve in serum-free media at 25 mg/mL, sterile-filter, aliquot, and store at –20°C for up to 1 month. Add to culture media 1:500 (v/v) as needed.

Dexamethasone stock (500X). Add 1 mL absolute ethanol per milligram, swirl to dissolve, and add 49 mL sterile serum-free medium per milliliter of ethanol for a final concentration of 20 μg/mL. Aliquot and store at –20°C. Add to culture media 1:500 (v/v) as needed.

MC3T3-E1 differentiation media. Add 50 mL fetal calf serum (FCS), 5 mL of 100X penicillin/streptomycin (P/S), 10 mL of 50X β-glycerolphosphate stock, 1 mL of 500X ascorbic acid stock, and 1 mL of 500X dexamethasone stock to 433 mL of alpha MEM.

4% Formaldehyde. Dilute formaldehyde solution, as supplied, to 4% in PBS.

13.7 Methods

13.7.1 Session 1: Prepare Hydrogels*

1. In a fume hood, mix acrylamide, bis-acrylamide, microspheres, and TEMED with sterile PBS in 15 mL conical tubes according to the recipes in Table 13.1.

2. Cap the tubes and vortex.

3. Degas the mixtures in a vacuum desiccator for 15 min. Removing oxygen from the solution speeds up polymerization and ensures more uniform polymerization:

   a. Loosen the cap of each conical tube approximately half a turn.

   b. Transfer the tubes to the desiccator and connect the vacuum line.

   c. Wait 15 min before removing the tubes.

4. Initiate polymerization of the PA mixtures one at a time so that they do not polymerize before you are finished making the hydrogels. Begin with the lowest PA concentration

---

* The hydrogels are prepared in a nonsterile environment and then UV sterilized prior to cell seeding.

TABLE 13.1

Recipes for Mixing Acrylamide and bis-Acrylamide to Generate Gels of Different Stiffness

Tube No.	Target Elastic Modulus	40% stock Acrylamide (μL)	2% Stock bis-acrylamide (μL)	TEMED (μL)	Microspheres (μL)	PBS (mL)
1	5 kPa	250	150	2	2	1.6
2	20 kPa	400	260	2	2	1.34
3	40 kPa	400	480	2	2	1.12

(tube no. 1) since it will take the longest to polymerize. *Note: Curved forceps with an extra fine, curved tip are helpful for handling the coverslips.*

a. Label four chlorosilanated glass slides for each gel stiffness. Lay them flat in a fume hood with the treated side up. *Note: At a minimum, you will need one hydrogel of each concentration for mechanical characterization and a second for cell seeding. Preparing four of each concentration will provide extras in case of breakage.*

b. In a fume hood, add 20 μL of APS to the first hydrogel mixture.

c. Quickly cap the solution and briefly vortex the polymerizing solution.

d. Quickly pipette 75 μL of the hydrogel solution onto the center of each of the four glass slides. Next, add the coverslip with the treated side down (Figure 13.2b). To prevent air bubbles from being trapped within the hydrogel, hold the coverslip approximately vertically, align the coverslip edge with the edge of the solution, and gently lower the coverslip, causing the hydrogel to spread beneath. The coverslip can be repositioned toward the center of the slide if needed.

e. Repeat steps 4b–4d for each PA mixture.

5. Allow the hydrogels to polymerize for 30 min or more. Monitor the unused solutions by tilting the tubes from side to side to determine when the hydrogels are fully polymerized. *Note: Fully polymerized gels may appear wet because excess PBS will accumulate around the gel.*

6. Carefully slide the coverslips and attached hydrogels off the glass slides. Place each coverslip–gel composite (gel side up) into one well of a new 12-well plate. Return the chlorosilanated slides to your instructor so they can be used again.

7. Rinse the hydrogels twice for 5 min in PBS to remove any unpolymerized acrylamide. The hydrogels should be stored in PBS and can be stored indefinitely at 4°C.

13.7.2 Session 2: Functionalize the Hydrogels with Collagen I

1. Remove and discard the PBS from the 12-well plates with the coverslip–gel composites.

2. Carefully move one hydrogel of each stiffness into a separate 12-well plate, rehydrate with PBS, and set aside for mechanical characterization in a subsequent lab session.

Note: It may be helpful in future lab sessions if you make a small mark on the bottom surface of the coverslip using a lab marker.

3. Activate the remaining nine hydrogels with sulfo-SANPAH:

   a. Add 500 μL of 0.2 mg/mL sulfo-SANPAH solution to each hydrogel surface. If 500 μL is not sufficient to cover the entire surface, add more.

   b. Place the hydrogels under the UV lamp (320–365 nm) for 10 min.

   c. Rinse each hydrogel twice with 1 mL 50 mM HEPES to remove excess sulfo-SANPAH.

   d. Dilute the 3 mg/mL stock collagen solution with 50 mM HEPES to a final concentration of 0.1 mg/mL and a final volume of 5 mL. To prevent the collagen from precipitating, add the HEPES gradually, vortexing between each addition.

   e. Add 500 μL of the collagen solution onto each hydrogel and incubate overnight at 37°C.

The following steps may be performed by an instructor in preparation for the next session:

1. Rinse each hydrogel with 5 mL PBS.

2. Remove the rinse and replace with 5 mL fresh PBS.

3. Repeat rinse a third time.

4. To sterilize the hydrogels, place the open plates under the UV light in a biosafety cabinet (BSC) for 60 min or more. The lids should be sterilized next to the plates.

5. Once the hydrogels are sterilized, they can be stored indefinitely in sterile PBS at 4°C.

13.7.3 Session 3: Seed Cells onto the Functionalized Hydrogels

1. In a 37°C water bath, warm MC3T3-E1 differentiation media and ~4 mL of trypsin.

2. Prepare the BSC for use by wiping it down with 70% ethanol and arranging necessary reagents and disposables. Place the 12-well plates containing the hydrogels in the BSC.

3. Prepare the MC3T3-E1 cells for seeding:

   a. Remove the cells from the incubator.

   b. View the cells under the microscope. Note the cell morphology and extent of confluence.

   c. Trypsinize the cells (refer to trypsinization protocol in Appendix 1), rinse once in media, and spin down.

   d. Resuspend the cells in 1 mL of differentiation media.

   e. Count the cells using a hemacytometer (refer to hemacytometer protocol in Appendix 2).

   f. Dilute the suspension to a final concentration of 0.2×10^6 cells/mL.

4. Remove the PBS from the hydrogels and replace with 1 mL of the cell suspension.

5. Place the hydrogels in the incubator and allow the cells to attach and grow 4–7 days with media changes every 2–3 days.

13.7.4 Session 4: Calibrate the Microscope's Fine-Focus Knob

Refer to Figure 13.3 for an illustration of the concepts involved in the following steps.

1. Obtain 10 or more coverslips. In your lab notebook, record the thickness of the coverslip as provided by the manufacturer.
2. Carefully draw a backslash (\) on the top surface of one coverslip with a lab marker and a slash (/) on the bottom surface of a second coverslip. Stack the coverslips so that the slashes make an X (Figure 13.4). *Note: It may be helpful to use differently colored markers.*

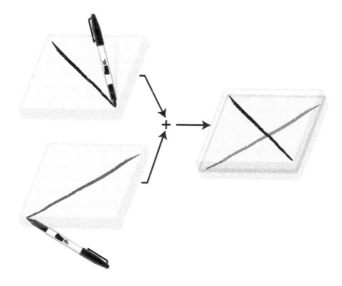

Figure 13.4

Schematic of the coverslip stack that will be used to quantify the relationship between turning the microscope's fine-focus knob and vertical movement of the focal point. This relationship will be used in the calculation of the stiffness of the PA gels. Using a high-powered objective, focus on the lower surface of the coverslip stack and record the position of the fine-focus knob. Next, find the focal plane of the top surface of the stack by turning only the fine-focus knob. Record the number of FFUs through which you rotated the knob as the focal plane moved from the bottom to the top of the stack of coverslips. Repeat this process after adding 1, 2, 3,...8 coverslips to the middle of the stack.

3. Place the coverslip stack on the stage of the microscope with the X approximately centered in the field of view. Ideally, both the slash and backslash will be visible in the same field of view.

4. Using the highest power objective available, focus on the slash (the lower surface of the bottom coverslip).

5. Record the position of the fine-focus knob in your lab book.

6. Turning only the fine-focus knob, find the focal plane of the backslash (the top surface of the top coverslip). Take note of which direction you must turn the fine-focus knob to move up through the glass.

7. Record the new position of the fine-focus knob. Determine and record the number of FFUs you rotated the knob through as the focal plane moved from the bottom to the top of the stack of coverslips.

8. Place a third coverslip in the middle of the stack and repeat the measurement.

9. Continuing adding coverslips, one at a time, and taking measurements until you have a stack of 10 coverslips.

13.7.5 Session 5: Characterize Hydrogel Dimensions and Material Properties

In this session, you will work with the hydrogels that were set aside and *not* functionalized with collagen or seeded with cells. There should be one hydrogel for each stiffness.

1. Set up the microscope for fluorescence imaging; use a filter cube compatible with the excitation and emission characteristics of the microspheres (EX: 505 nm, EM: 515 nm). Allow the lamp to warm up ~15 min.

2. Measure the thickness of the first hydrogel:

   a. Fill a small petri dish about halfway with PBS.

   b. Place one hydrogel in the dish, making sure it is resting on the bottom.

   c. Place the dish on the stage of the microscope and bring the hydrogel into focus.

   d. Switch to the highest power objective available, use fluorescence illumination, and scan the depth of the hydrogel to verify that the microspheres are embedded throughout.

   e. Identify one or more microspheres at the very lowest point in the hydrogel. This is the interface between the hydrogel and underlying coverslip. You should be able to move the focal plane *down* from this position to see the bottom of the coverslip (and, if applicable, the mark you left in Session 2). Return to the lowest point in the hydrogel and focus carefully on one microsphere. *Note: The measurements in this lab require patience and precision. At this point, it is helpful to train your eye to identify when the microsphere of interest is exactly in focus.*

   f. Record the position of the fine-focus knob in your lab book.

    g. Slowly turn the fine-focus knob to move the focal plane up through the hydrogel, keeping track of the number of revolutions made, until a microsphere at the highest point of the hydrogel is in focus.

    h. Record the number of FFUs required to move from the lowest point to the highest point in the hydrogel. FFUs will be converted to microns using the calibration curve generated in Session 4.

    i. Repeat the thickness measurement in two additional locations within the same hydrogel.

3. Measure the stiffness of the first hydrogel:

    a. Carefully drop a single steel microball near the center of the hydrogel.

    b. Using transmitted light, center the ball in the field of view.

    c. Using fluorescence, focus on a microsphere at the hydrogel surface and directly under the center of the ball. If no microsphere is suitably positioned, move the ball to a nearby location.

    d. Note the position of the fine-focus knob in your lab notebook and study the pattern of microspheres around the microsphere of interest.

    e. Without touching the microscope or moving the hydrogel *at all,* remove the ball by holding a magnet above the hydrogel.

    f. Verify that the field of view is unchanged and bring the microsphere of interest back into focus. Record the number of FFUs between the microsphere's deformed and undeformed positions.

    g. Repeat the stiffness measurement five times.

4. Repeat steps 2 and 3 for one hydrogel of each stiffness.

13.7.6 Session 6: Stain Cells with von Kossa's Method

1. After 4–7 days in culture, remove the hydrogels from the incubator. It is not necessary to keep the samples sterile from this point forward.

2. Stain gels using the von Kossa method:

    a. Aspirate the media out of each well and replace with 4% formaldehyde in PBS. Treat for 15 min at room temperature (RT).

    b. Rinse each gel twice with 4 mL dH_2O.

    c. Add 1 mL 5% silver nitrate to each well and place the hydrogels under a UV light source for 30 min.

    d. Rinse each gel twice with 4 mL dH_2O.

    e. Add 1 mL 5% sodium thiosulfate to each well and treat for 3 min.

    f. Rinse each gel twice with 4 mL dH_2O.

3. Use transmitted light microscopy and a low powered objective to capture *representative* micrographs of each gel. The cytoplasm will appear pink and phosphate deposits will appear black. For comparison, take several images of the cells on the glass slide surrounding the gels. *Note: Phosphate deposits may be viewed more easily without phase contrast.*

TABLE 13.2
Suggested Format for Presenting Gel Deformation Data

	Individual Displacement Measurements (μm)					Mean Displacement ± SD (μm)	Mean Stiffness ± SD (kPa)
	1	2	3	4	5		
5 kPA Gel							
20 kPA Gel							
40 kPA Gel							

4. Obtain a calibration image so that you will be able to add a scale bar to representative micrographs when documenting your results. You may get a calibration image from your instructor or acquire an image of a stage micrometer or hemacytometer grid using the same magnification as in the micrographs.

13.8 Data Processing and Reporting

Briefly report the results of your experiment in paragraph and graphical form. Each of the key results to report in text, figure, and/or table format is described next.

1. Include a graph of the microscope calibration data illustrating the relationship between FFUs and vertical distance traveled by the objective (x-axis: FFUs; y-axis: distance). Display the equation of the best-fit line, fit through the origin, and the corresponding r^2 value on the graph. Within the text, report the conversion factor used to translate FFUs to microns for determination of the hydrogel properties.

2. Report the mean and standard deviation of the measured hydrogel thicknesses. Comment on the variability in the measurements within a single gel and between gels of different stiffness.

3. Construct a table, similar to Table 13.2, of the deformation data and hydrogel stiffness. Briefly describe each calculation in the text.

4. In one professional-quality figure with multiple panels, include at least one representative micrograph of the von Kossa stained samples for each gel stiffness. Include a scale bar. Summarize your observations within the text.

13.9 Prelab Questions

1. Calculate the percent weight by volume (w/v) of the acrylamide and bis-acrylamide solutions just prior to polymerization

2.
   a. Calculate the volumes of the stock collagen (3 mg/mL) and HEPES (50 mM) needed to make 5 mL of 0.1 mg/mL collagen in HEPES.
   b. What is the final concentration of HEPES in the diluted collagen solution?

TABLE 13.3
Sample Data for Displacement of an Embedded Microsphere

Actual		Measured		Relative Error	
d (m)	E (Pa)	$d + \Delta d$ (m)	$E + \Delta E$ (Pa)	$\Delta d/d$ (%)	$\Delta E/E$ (%)
36.4×10^{-6}	5,000	38.2×10^{-6}		5	
36.4×10^{-6}	5,000	40.0×10^{-6}		10	
36.4×10^{-6}	5,000	32.7×10^{-6}		−10	
9.10×10^{-6}	40,000	9.55×10^{-6}		5	
9.10×10^{-6}	40,000	10.0×10^{-6}		10	
9.10×10^{-6}	40,000	8.19×10^{-6}		−10	

c. What is the *maximum possible* density (milligrams per square centimeter) of collagen on the PA gel surface that could result from the protocol used? State any conditions that would need to be met in order to achieve this maximum density.

3. On which PA substrate do you think the MC3T3-E1 cells will express a more osteoblast-like phenotype? Briefly explain your answer and cite references used to gather evidence to support your hypothesis.

4. There will be error associated with measuring the displacement of the microsphere when characterizing the stiffness of the hydrogels (Damljanovic et al. 2005). One source of error is associated with finding the correct focal plane for a microsphere both before and after deformation. A second source of error is in the selection of the appropriate microsphere to track—specifically, a microsphere directly below the lowest point on the ball.

a. The modulus measured experimentally is equal to the true modulus (E) plus a small amount of error (ΔE). Calculate the percent error in the measured modulus ($\Delta E/E$) that would occur as a result of errors in measured microsphere displacement (Δd) for the sample data in Table 13.3. Assume that $v = 0.3$, $r = 0.5$ mm, $\rho_b = 8000$ kg/m^3, and $\rho_f = 1000$ kg/m^3.

b. Is the percent error in the modulus dependent on the Poisson ratio? Ball radius? Fluid density? Ball density?

c. Compared to the actual value, would the calculated modulus be *higher, lower,* or *the same* if you mistakenly tracked a microsphere in contact with the ball somewhere other than at its lowest point? Briefly explain your answer.

13.10 Postlab Questions

1. The density of cross-links within a PA gel determines its stiffness. Cross-link density may also affect surface chemistry and, as a result, ligand density. Briefly describe an experiment that could be performed to test the hypothesis that ligand density, rather than stiffness, is primarily influencing cell differentiation in this experiment.

2. An observable change in cell phenotype is the result of an underlying change in gene expression. To affect gene expression, an extracellular signal, such as substrate stiffness, must travel a complex path across the cell membrane and through the cell interior. The transduction pathway may be mechanical, biochemical, or a combination of both.

Research the mechanisms by which cells transduce mechanical signals, list at least five molecules involved in this process, and provide a one-sentence description of each.

3. Find another example in the literature where substrate stiffness was used to influence cell differentiation. Briefly describe the methods used and findings of this study, emphasizing the similarities and differences compared to the current experiment.

4. A classic tensile test provides an alternate to the "microball" method for measuring gel stiffness. Calculate the final gauge length of "dog bone" specimens (with moduli of 5, 20, and 40 kPa), initially with a gauge length of 10 mm and cross-sectional area of 12 mm², after a 1 g weight is attached. Assume that all tests are within the linear region of the stress–strain curve and the specimens remain hydrated during the test.

References

Alberts, B., A. Johnson, J. Lewis, M. Raff, K. Roberts, and P. Walter. 2007. *Molecular biology of the cell,* 5th ed. New York: Garland Science.

Beningo, K. A., C. M. Lo, and Y. L. Wang. 2002. Flexible polyacrylamide substrata for the analysis of mechanical interactions at cell-substratum adhesions. *Methods in Cell Biology* 69:325–339.

Bonewald, L. F., S. E. Harris, J. Rosser, M. R. Dallas, S. L. Dallas, N. P. Camacho, B. Boyan, and A. Boskey. 2003. von Kossa staining alone is not sufficient to confirm that mineralization in vitro represents bone formation. *Calcified Tissue International* 72 (5): 537–547.

Damljanovic, V., B. C. Lagerholm, and K. Jacobson. 2005. Bulk and micropatterned conjugation of extracellular matrix proteins to characterized polyacrylamide substrates for cell mechanotransduction assays. *BioTechniques* 39 (6): 847–851.

Discher, D. E., P. Janmey, and Y. L. Wang. 2005. Tissue cells feel and respond to the stiffness of their substrate. *Science* 310 (5751): 1139–1143.

Engler, A., L. Bacakova, C. Newman, A. Hategan, M. Griffin, and D. Discher. 2004. Substrate compliance versus ligand density in cell on gel responses. *Biophysical Journal* 86 (1 Pt 1): 617–628.

Engler, A. J., S. Sen, H. L. Sweeney, and D. E. Discher. 2006. Matrix elasticity directs stem cell lineage specification. *Cell* 126 (4): 677–689.

Fung, Y. 1993. *Biomechanics: Mechanical properties of living tissues.* New York: Springer–Verlag.

Johnson, K. L. 1987. *Contact mechanics.* Cambridge, England: Cambridge University Press.

Khatiwala, C. B., S. R. Peyton, and A. J. Putnam. 2006. Intrinsic mechanical properties of the extracellular matrix affect the behavior of pre-osteoblastic MC3T3-E1 cells. *American Journal of Physiology. Cell Physiology* 290 (6): C1640–C1650.

Pelham, R. J., Jr., and Y. Wang. 1997. Cell locomotion and focal adhesions are regulated by substrate flexibility. *Proceedings of National Academy of Sciences USA* 94 (25): 13661–13665.

Tse, J. R., and A. J. Engler. 2010. Preparation of hydrogel substrates with tunable mechanical properties. *Current Protocols in Cell Biology* June Chapter 10:Unit 10.16.

Chapter **14**

Effect of Culture Configuration (Two versus Three Dimensions) on Matrix Accumulation

14.1 Background

Like many connective tissues, articular cartilage has an extensive extracellular matrix (ECM) that imparts material properties critical for the tissue's function. In patients suffering from osteoarthritis, the cartilage ECM degrades and the patient experiences joint pain. Investigational approaches to treating osteoarthritis include growing cartilaginous tissue in the lab and using this engineered tissue to resurface the damaged joint. A significant challenge of cartilage tissue engineering is producing a matrix similar in structure and content to native cartilage in an efficient and reproducible manner.

The ECM of cartilage is primarily composed of aggrecan and collagen type II. Aggrecan is a huge proteoglycan consisting of over 100 polysaccharide chains, called glycosaminoglycans (GAGs), attached to a protein core (Alberts et al. 2007). The specific GAG chains found in aggrecan are chondroitin sulfate and keratan sulfate (Alberts et al. 2007). Individual aggrecan monomers are immobilized within cartilage on a backbone of hyaluronan, creating huge aggregates that contribute to the compressive properties of the tissue (Figure 14.1) (Mow and Huiskes 2005). Collagen II forms an extensive fibrillar network throughout the ECM to provide the tissue's tensile strength (Mow and Huiskes 2005). Chondrocytes are specialized cells that sparsely populate articular cartilage and maintain tissue homeostasis through synthesis, organization, and remodeling of these and other ECM components.

Long-term culture of chondrocytes on a biomaterial scaffold allows for accumulation of cartilaginous matrix and the formation of a cohesive tissue construct

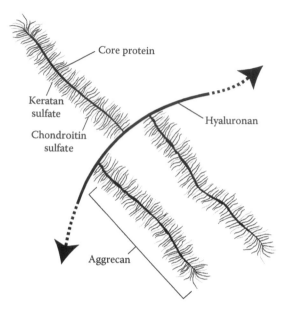

Figure 14.1

A schematic showing three aggrecan monomers attached to a hyaluronan backbone to form a portion of an aggrecan aggregate. Each aggrecan monomer is composed of a core protein with many keratan sulfate and chondroitin sulfate side chains.

(Hunziker et al. 2006). Cartilage-like constructs have also been formed without the use of a scaffold by preculturing chondrocytes within a natural hydrogel called alginate. Chondrocytes can be recovered from alginate culture with a cell-associated matrix and these alginate-recovered cells form a cohesive cartilaginous tissue in subsequent culture (Masuda et al. 2003). To engineer a cartilage tissue equivalent, either with or without a scaffold, cells must synthesize and deposit the appropriate ECM. The degree to which cells retain this newly synthesized ECM depends on the environment in which they are grown; therefore, a culture configuration that produces the desired result must be used. This experiment will compare two different culture systems—two-dimensional (2-D) monolayer and three-dimensional (3-D) alginate culture—to determine which favors retention of GAGs produced by chondrocytes.

Accumulation of GAG produced by chondrocytes is commonly measured using a dye called dimethylmethylene blue (DMMB) (Farndale, Buttle, and Barrett 1986). DMMB selectively binds to sulfated GAGs, such as the chondroitin sulfate and keratan sulfate side chains of aggrecan, causing a shift in absorbance to a maximum of 525 nm. Absorbance at 525 nm (A_{525}) is measured using a spectrophotometer and compared to A_{525} of standard solutions to determine the concentration of sulfated GAG in a solution. The amount of GAG recovered from monolayer and alginate cultures will be compared by digesting the cultures and subsequently performing a DMMB assay on the digests. GAG content will be normalized to the number of cells present in the culture prior to digestion. Cell content will be quantified using a DNA assay called PicoGreen®, which is discussed more extensively in Appendix 3.

14.2 Learning Objectives

The objectives of this experiment are to

- Establish 3-D cultures by encapsulating bovine chondrocytes in alginate, a natural hydrogel commonly used as a biomaterial
- Learn to perform widely applicable assays to measure GAG and DNA while gaining experience operating a spectrophotometer and fluorometer
- Using statistics, compare GAG accumulation in 3-D and 2-D chondrocyte cultures to investigate the significance of culture conditions in tissue-engineering applications

14.3 Overview of Experiment

This experiment involves establishing 2-D monolayer and 3-D alginate cultures of bovine chondrocytes. The cultures will be maintained for a week or longer to allow the chondrocytes to synthesize and secrete ECM molecules, including GAGs. After the cultures are terminated, the recovered cells and associated ECM are enzymatically digested with proteinase-K. The digests will be assayed to measure total GAG and DNA content using the DMMB and PicoGreen assays, respectively. The two culture methods will be compared to determine which results in the higher GAG accumulation *per cell*.

14.4 Safety Notes

Place a small biohazard sharps container in the biosafety cabinet (BSC) so that contaminated needles can be thrown away immediately after use. Do not attempt to recap or remove the needle from the syringe after use. Use good lab practices and review all relevant MSDSs.

14.5 Materials

In addition to the general equipment and supplies, the following are needed to complete this experiment:

14.5.1 Reagents and Consumables

- >3 × 10^6 Chondrocytes in suspension
- Trypan blue
- Chondrocyte media (recipe follows)
- Sterile 12 mg/mL alginate in 0.9% NaCl

- Sterile 102 mM CaCl$_2$
- Sterile 3 cc syringe
- 20-Gauge needle
- Sterile 55 mM sodium citrate in 0.9% NaCl
- Phosphate-buffered EDTA (PBE)
- 50X Proteinase-K (25 mg/mL in PBE)
- PicoGreen dsDNA assay kit (including TE buffer and 100 µg/mL DNA standard; Molecular Probes)
- 10 mg/mL Chondroitin sulfate sodium salt from shark cartilage in PBE (GAG standard)
- Dimethylmethylene blue (DMMB) dye
- Glycine
- Filter paper
- Sterile spatula
- Untreated 25 cm^2 culture flask
- Tissue culture treated 12.5 cm^2 flask
- Untreated flat-bottom, 96-well plate

14.5.2 Equipment and Supplies

- Sterile beaker (containing a stir bar and covered with foil)
- Promega Quanti-Fluor fluorometer (EX: 480 nm, EM: 520 nm) with minicell cuvettes
- Amber storage bottle
- Microplate reader (to measure absorbance at 525 nm) with acquisition software

14.6 Recipes

250X l-Proline stock (100 mM). Dissolve 0.46 g l-proline in 40 mL DMEM/F12, filter through a 0.2 µm filter, pipette 2 mL aliquots into sterile cryovials, and store at –20°C.

Chondrocyte media. Add 50 mL fetal bovine serum (FBS), 5 mL of 100X penicillin/ streptomycin (P/S), 2 mL of 250X l-proline stock, 5 mL of 200 mM l-glutamine, and 5 mL of 10 mM nonessential amino acids to 433 mL DMEM/F12.

1X PBS. Add 50 mL 10X PBS (with Ca^{2+} and Mg^{2+}) to 400 mL deionized H$_2$O (dH$_2$O). Mix well, adjust pH to 7.4 with HCl and NaOH, bring total volume to 500 mL with dH$_2$O, and either sterile-filter through a 0.2 µm filter or autoclave.

0.9% Sodium chloride (NaCl). Dissolve NaCl in dH$_2$O at 9 mg/mL.

12 mg/mL Alginate. Weigh out 1.2 g alginate in an autoclavable bottle, add 100 mL 0.9% NaCl, mix with a magnetic stir plate until dissolved (>2 h), autoclave, aliquot, and store at 4°C.

102 mM Calcium chloride (CaCl$_2$). Dissolve CaCl$_2$ dihydrate (MW = 147) in dH$_2$O at 15 mg/mL, adjust pH to 7.1 with HCl and NaOH, autoclave, and store at room temperature (RT).

55 m*M* Sodium citrate. Dissolve sodium citrate dihydrate (MW = 294) at 16.2 mg/mL in 0.9% NaCl, adjust pH to 7.1 with HCl and NaOH, autoclave, and store at RT.

0.1 *M* Phosphate buffer. Reconstitute according to manufacturer's instructions or purchase 1X solution.

PBE. Dissolve ethylenediaminetetraacetic acid disodium salt dihydrate (EDTA; MW = 372) at 1.86 mg/mL in 0.1 *M* phosphate buffer, adjust pH to 7.1 with HCl and NaOH, and store at RT.

50X Proteinase-K stock. Dilute proteinase-K in PBE to a concentration of 25 mg/mL, prepare 100 μL aliquots, and store at –20°C for up to a year. This is a 50X stock solution. Dilute the stock in PBE as needed.

1X TE buffer. Dilute the 20X TE buffer supplied with the PicoGreen kit in dH$_2$O.

100 μg/mL DNA standard. Prepare 5 μL aliquots of the DNA standard provided with the PicoGreen kit. Store at –20°C.

PicoGreen. Prepare 5 μL aliquots of the 200X solution provided with the PicoGreen kit. Store at –20°C.

10 mg/mL GAG standard. Dissolve chondroitin sulfate from shark cartilage in PBE at 10 mg/mL, prepare 100 μL aliquots, and store at –20°C.

DMMB dye. Dissolve 0.8 mg DMMB in 1 mL ethanol, wrap tube in aluminum foil, and dissolve overnight with stirring. Prepare 1 L of 40 m*M* NaCl + 40 m*M* glycine. Bring DMMB to 500 mL in NaCl/glycine solution, pH 3.0, and filter into an amber bottle. Check the absorbance of the DMMB solution at 525 nm using the NaCl/glycine solution as a blank. If the absorbance is >0.32, add more NaCl/glycine solution. Store up to 3 months at 25°C.

14.7 Methods

14.7.1 Session 1: Initiate the Cultures

1. Warm chondrocyte media in a 37°C water bath.
2. Prepare the BSC for use by wiping it down with 70% ethanol and arranging necessary reagents and disposables.
3. Determine the density of the cell suspension:
   a. Collect two sterile samples of the cell suspension provided by your instructor.
   b. Count the cells using a hemacytometer (refer to hemacytometer protocol in Appendix 2).
   c. Adjust the cell concentration to 1×10^6 cells/mL. *Note: You will need at least 3 mL of the cell suspension to complete the lab.*
4. Establish a high-density monolayer culture by adding 1.25 mL of the cell suspension and 1.25 mL of chondrocyte media to a *tissue culture treated* T12.5 flask. Place the flask in the incubator.
5. Make the cell-seeded alginate beads (Figure 14.2):
   a. Transfer 1.75 mL of the cell suspension to a new 15 mL conical tube.

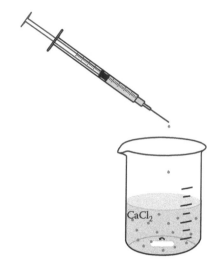

Figure 14.2
Cells suspended in alginate are ejected dropwise from a syringe into a calcium chloride ($CaCl_2$) bath. Calcium chloride polymerizes the alginate, encapsulating the cells within each alginate bead.

    b.   Spin the cells down, using a counterbalance, at 300 g for 5 min and discard the supernatant.

    c.   Use a serological pipette to add 1.75 mL sterile alginate solution to the tube containing the cell pellet.

    d.   Using the same pipette, gently mix the cell suspension by slowly drawing the solution up and down, being careful not to create bubbles. The cells should be uniformly distributed in the alginate at a density of 1×10^6 cells/mL.

    e.   Add 25 mL sterile $CaCl_2$ solution to a sterile beaker containing a stir bar.

    f.   Lightly spray a magnetic stir plate with ethanol and place it in the center of the BSC. Connect the power cord.

    g.   Place the beaker on the stir plate and set at a slow speed (fast speeds will create tear-drop shaped beads).

    h.   Use a 3 cc syringe with a 20-gauge needle to draw up 1.25 mL of the alginate/cell solution, making as few bubbles as possible.

    i.   Hold the needle over the beaker such that the body of the needle is at a 45° angle to the surface of the $CaCl_2$ solution. The opening of the needle should face toward you.

    j.   Slowly push in the plunger of the syringe to eject about two drops of alginate per second into the $CaCl_2$ solution. This speed will ensure that the alginate will leave the syringe quickly enough that the cells will not clump at the bottom of the syringe.

    k.   Discard the empty syringe in a biohazardous sharps container.

    l.   Let the alginate beads sit in the $CaCl_2$ for 5 min.

  6. Rinse the alginate beads:

    a.   Carefully aspirate the $CaCl_2$. Use a 10 mL pipette pushed straight down onto the base of the beaker to avoid damaging or aspirating any beads. *Do not use a Pasteur pipette.*

    b.   Add 25 mL sterile PBS and allow the beads to sit for 5 min.

    c.   Repeat the rinse two more times.

7. Establish the alginate cultures:

    a.   Carefully aspirate the PBS rinse from the beads.

    b.   Using a sterile spatula, transfer the beads to an *untreated* T25 flask. Using an untreated flask inhibits the growth of cells that may "escape" from the alginate beads during culture.

    c.   Add 2.5 mL chondrocyte media to the flask.

    d.   Place the flask in the incubator.

8. Carefully remove the monolayer culture from the incubator and view using a light microscope. Summarize your observations about the morphology, density, etc., of the cells in your lab notebook and take a representative image of the cells. Repeat with the alginate cultures.

9. Culture the cells for at least 1 week with media changes every 2–3 days.

14.7.2 Session 2: Terminate the Cultures

1. Warm a water bath to 50°C.

2. View the cells in monolayer and alginate culture using a light microscope. Summarize your observations about the morphology, density, etc., of the cells in your lab notebook and take a representative image of the cells in each culture condition using a high magnification.

3. Obtain a calibration image so that you will be able to add a scale bar to representative micrographs when documenting your results. You may get a calibration image from your instructor or acquire an image of a stage micrometer or hemacytometer grid using the same magnification as in the micrographs.

4. Make a 0.5 mg/mL proteinase-K solution by combining 100 μL of the 50X stock solution with 4.9 mL PBE.

5. Aspirate and discard the media from the monolayer culture. *Note: This step and subsequent steps do not need to be performed in a BSC.*

6. Add 2 mL of proteinase-K to the T12.5 flask, cap the flask, and place it in a 50°C water bath on a rack above the water level. Make sure that the flask is flat so that the entire cell monolayer is covered with proteinase-K.

7. Dissolve the alginate beads:

    a.   Aspirate the media from the alginate bead culture using a 10 mL pipette pushed straight down onto the base of the flask to avoid damaging or aspirating any beads.

    b.   Add 5 mL of sodium citrate to the flask.

    c.   Gently shake the flask as the beads disassociate.

    d.   After ~10 min, once all the beads have disappeared, transfer the solution to a conical tube.

    e.   Spin the cells down, using a counterbalance, at 300 g for 5 min, gently aspirate, and discard the supernatant.

    f.   Resuspend the cells in 5 mL of sodium citrate to dissolve any residual alginate.

g. Spin the cells down, using a counterbalance, at 300 g for 5 min, gently aspirate, and discard the supernatant.

h. Rinse the cells with 10 mL of PBS.

i. Spin the cells down, using a counterbalance, at 300 g for 5 min, gently aspirate, and discard the supernatant.

j. Add 2 mL of proteinase-K to the cell pellet.

8. Retrieve the T12.5 flask from the water bath, confirm that the cell monolayer has been released from the flask, and transfer the digest to a conical tube.

9. Tightly cap the conical tubes containing the alginate-recovered and monolayer-recovered cells and place them in a 50°C water bath.

10. Digest the cells overnight and store the samples at –20°C until they are needed for the DMMB and PicoGreen assays. *Note: Your instructor may perform this step for you.*

14.7.3 Session 3: Measure Glycosaminoglycan Content of the Culture Digests

1. Turn on and configure the absorbance plate reader to measure absorbance at 525 nm (A_{525}).

2. Remove the GAG standards and the samples (alginate-recovered and monolayer-recovered cell digests) from the freezer and allow them to thaw at RT.

3. Prepare the GAG standards (125 to 0 µg/mL) in duplicate as described in the DMMB protocol (Appendix 4).

4. Load the standards and samples (in duplicate) into a multiwell plate as described in the DMMB protocol. *Note: It is very important to vortex each sample.*

5. Measure and record A_{525} for each standard and sample. If any sample is out of range of the standards or the spectrophotometer detection limit, dilute the sample more and repeat the measurement until the reading falls within the working range of the calibration curve. Make careful notes regarding the dilutions in your lab notebook.

6. Add your raw data for standards and samples to the class database that the instructor has created (e.g., Excel spreadsheet on lab computer). Save the file. These data will be shared with all members of the class.

7. Store the remaining alginate-recovered and monolayer-recovered cell digests at –20°C for the next session.

14.7.4 Session 4: Measure DNA Content of the Culture Digests

1. Turn on and configure the fluorometer to excite at ~480 nm and measure emission at ~520 nm.

2. Remove two 5 µL PicoGreen aliquots, the DNA standards, and the samples (alginate-recovered and monolayer-recovered cells) from the freezer and allow them to thaw at RT.

3. Prepare the PicoGreen dye solution as described in the PicoGreen protocol (Appendix 3).

4. Prepare the DNA standards (100 to 0 ng DNA/mL final volume) as described in the PicoGreen protocol.

5. Generate a standard curve for the DNA assay. If the standard curve is not linear, try to identify the source of error and repeat until a reliable standard curve is obtained.

6. Prepare duplicate samples for the DNA assay. For this particular experiment, mixing 10 µL of each sample with 240 µL TE buffer should yield a concentration within the range of the standards. *Note: It is very important to vortex each sample before and after diluting it.*

7. Perform the PicoGreen assay to measure the DNA concentration in each sample. If any sample is out of range of the standards or the fluorometer detection limit, dilute the sample more and repeat the measurement until the reading falls within the working range of the calibration curve. Make careful notes regarding the dilutions in your lab notebook.

8. Add your raw data for standards and samples to the class database that the instructor has created (e.g., Excel spreadsheet on lab computer). Save the file. These data will be shared with all members of the class.

14.8 Data Processing and Reporting

Briefly report the results of your experiment in paragraph and graphical form. Each of the key results to report in text, figure, and/or table format is described next.

1. Include representative images of cells within the flask and alginate beads. Comment on cell morphology and other distinguishing features.

2. Include a graph of the GAG standard curve (x-axis: GAG concentration; y-axis: absorbance). Display the equation of the best-fit polynomial and the corresponding r^2 value on the graph.

3. Include a table, similar to Table 14.1, displaying the raw data and subsequent calculations from the DMMB assay. Briefly describe each calculation in the text.

4. Include a graph of the DNA standard curve (x-axis: DNA concentration; y-axis: fluorescence). Display the equation of the best-fit line and the corresponding r^2 value on the graph.

5. Include a table, similar to Table 14.2, displaying the raw data and subsequent calculations from the PicoGreen assay. Briefly describe each calculation in the text. *Note: The DNA content of a bovine chondrocyte is 7.7 pg per chondrocyte (Kim et al. 1988).*

6. From the DNA content of your samples, calculate the total number of cells in culture at the time the culture was terminated. Comment on how these measurements compare to each other and to the number of cells used to initiate the cultures.

7. Report the amount of GAG retained per cell for each culture condition (2-D vs. 3-D).

8. Combine your data with data collected by your classmates. Generate a bar graph that displays the average GAG accumulation per cell for the two culture conditions. Include error bars corresponding to the standard deviation.

TABLE 14.1
Suggested Format for Reporting Data Collected from the DMMB Assay

	Sample Description	
	2-D Culture Digest	3-D Culture Digest
Absorbance		
Absorbance of duplicate		
Mean absorbance		
Difference in duplicates (percentage)		
GAG in sample (micrograms/milliliter)[a]		
Total GAG in sample		

[a] Calculate from the average absorbance and the standard curve.

TABLE 14.2
Suggested Format for Reporting Data Collected from the DNA Assay

	Sample Description	
	2-D Culture Digest	3-D Culture Digest
Fluorescence		
Fluorescence of duplicate		
Mean fluorescence		
Difference in duplicates (percentage)		
(DNA) in cuvette[a] (picograms/milliliter)		
Dilution factor[b]		
(DNA) in sample (picograms/milliliter)		
(Cells) in sample (cells/milliliter)		
Total cells in sample		

[a] Calculate from the average fluorescence and the standard curve.
[b] Dilution factor = total volume in cuvette ÷ volume of undiluted sample in cuvette.

9. Statistical analysis: use a t-test to determine if culture condition (2-D vs. 3-D) significantly affected GAG accumulation per cell. Report the sample size, degrees of freedom, critical t-value corresponding to $p < 0.05$, the p-value obtained from your data, and the statistical power.

14.9 Prelab Questions

1. According to the protocol for session 1, you should place the newly formed alginate beads in the incubator and image the monolayer culture using the microscope first. Why not image the alginate cultures first since you have them handy?

2. Chondrocytes embedded in alginate demonstrate a significant change in size and gene expression following sudden changes in osmolarity (Hung et al. 2003). These findings suggest that osmolarity may be an influence on extracellular matrix synthesis and accumulation.

   a. Calculate the osmolarity of the sodium chloride and calcium chloride used in the cell isolation protocol. Assume complete dissociation.

   b. What volume change do you expect when moving a cell from PBS, which has the same osmolarity as 0.9% sodium chloride, to media with an osmolarity of 360 mOsm? Report your answer as a percentage change relative to the initial cell volume. State any assumptions you make and verify that the calculation agrees with what is expected physiologically.

   c. Experimentally, changes in the 2-D projection of a cell's volume are easier to measure than changes in volume (e.g., cell area as viewed under a microscope). Calculate the percentage change in projected cell area associated with the volume change in part (b). State any assumptions you make.

   d. Use the model developed in parts (b) and (c) to calculate the change in cell area expected when you move a cell from a 360 mOsm solution to a 580 mOsm solution. How does this theoretical value compare with the experiment data previously reported (Hung et al. 2003)? If it is different, propose a hypothesis that may explain the discrepancy.

   e. Briefly discuss how regulating osmolarity may be a useful tool for cartilage tissue engineering.

3. Chondroitin sulfate is one of the side chains on the cartilage proteoglycan aggrecan and is widely used as a natural supplement to treat knee pain. A multicenter trial was conducted to determine the efficacy of chondroitin sulfate in relieving knee pain associated with osteoarthritis (OA). Review the report by Sawitzke and colleagues (2010) summarizing findings from the first 2 years of the study:

   a. Identify and describe as needed the following key components of the experimental design: null hypothesis, experimental groups, sample size, and the primary outcome measure.

   b. Summarize the major findings of the study.

   c. What was the approximate magnitude of the placebo effect in this study? What factor(s) may contribute to the placebo effect?

14.10 Postlab Questions

1. Your data likely show that chondrocytes can be recovered from alginate with more associated GAGs than those cultured in monolayer. Should this result be interpreted to conclude that monolayer cells do not produce GAGs? Explain your answer.

2. Compare and contrast this experiment's methods and results with those reported in Figure 2 of "A Novel Two-Step Method for the Formation of Tissue-Engineering Cartilage by Mature Chondrocytes: The Alginate-Recovered-Chondrocyte (ARC) Method" by Masuda and colleagues (2003). How were our methods different? How might these differences affect the results? For comparison with the published data, assume 7.7 pg DNA/chondrocyte.

3. Porous microcarrier beads are small spheres, typically less than a millimeter in diameter, that cells attach to and infiltrate. When used in conjunction with a stirred tank bioreactor, microcarrier beads allow compact culture of a large number of anchorage-dependent cells. Consider a microcarrier with the same external dimensions as an alginate bead and an extensive network of 75 μm diameter pores. Is a cell growing within the interior of the microcarrier in a 3-D culture environment? Briefly explain your answer.

References

Alberts, B., A. Johnson, J. Lewis, M. Raff, K. Roberts, and P. Walter. 2007. *Molecular biology of the cell,* 5th ed. New York: Garland Science.

Farndale, R. W., D. J. Buttle, and A. J. Barrett. 1986. Improved quantitation and discrimination of sulfated glycosaminoglycans by use of dimethylmethylene blue. *Biochimica et Biophysica Acta* 883 (2): 173–177.

Hung, C. T., M. A. LeRoux, G. D. Palmer, P. H. Chao, S. Lo, and W. B. Valhmu. 2003. Disparate aggrecan gene expression in chondrocytes subjected to hypotonic and hypertonic loading in 2D and 3D culture. *Biorheology* 40 (1–3): 61–72.

Hunziker, E., M. Spector, J. Libera, A. Gertzman, S. L. Woo, A. Ratcliffe, M. Lysaght, A. Coury, D. Kaplan, and G. Vunjak-Novakovic. 2006. Translation from research to applications. *Tissue Engineering* 12 (12): 3341–3364.

Kim, Y. J., R. L. Sah, J. Y. Doong, and A. J. Grodzinsky. 1988. Fluorometric assay of DNA in cartilage explants using Hoechst 33258. *Analytical Biochemistry* 174 (1): 168–176.

Masuda, K., R. L. Sah, M. J. Hejna, and E. J. Thonar. 2003. A novel two-step method for the formation of tissue-engineered cartilage by mature bovine chondrocytes: The alginate-recovered-chondrocyte (ARC) method. *Journal of Orthopaedic Research: Official Publication of the Orthopaedic Research Society* 21 (1): 139–148.

Mow, V. C., and R. Huiskes. 2005. *Basic orthopaedic biomechanics and mechano-biology.* Philadelphia: Lippincott Williams & Wilkins.

Sawitzke, A. D., H. Shi, M. F. Finco, D. D. Dunlop, C. L. Harris, N. G. Singer, J. D. Bradley, et al. 2010. Clinical efficacy and safety of glucosamine, chondroitin sulfate, their combination, celecoxib or placebo taken to treat osteoarthritis of the knee: 2-year results from GAIT. *Annals of the Rheumatic Diseases* 69 (8): 1459–1464.

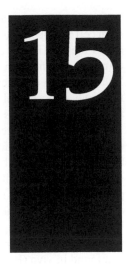

Combining In Silico and In Vitro Techniques to Engineer Pluripotent Stem Cell Fate

15.1 Background

Stem cells balance the capacity for sustained self-renewal with the potential to differentiate along specific tissue lineages. Successful use of stem cells for tissue engineering and regenerative medicine applications requires that precise control over this capacity be attained. However, robust control of stem cell fate has yet to be achieved and methodologies for maintaining stem cells outside the body or for their controlled differentiation into functional cells are still under development.

Stem cell bioengineering is focused on the quantitative description of the processes regulating stem cell fate and the use of this information for the development of clinically and industrially relevant cell-based technologies (Zandstra 2004). Realizing this goal requires a combination of in vitro, in vivo, and in silico approaches to elucidate the temporal and spatial regulatory mechanisms that underlie stem cell fate determination (Davey and Zandstra 2004). To date, stem cell bioengineering initiatives have studied the growth of cells on modified surfaces and culture configurations, methods to control medium supplementation and microenvironmental conditions, tools for primary cell manipulation, and quantitative measurement of primary cell responses, as well as mathematical models of cell population and individual cell processes (Zandstra 2004).

Mouse embryonic stem cells (mESCs) represent one major type of pluripotent population derived from the inner cell mass (ICM) of the early embryo (Martin 1981; Evans and Kaufman 1981), and they are commonly used in the tissue-engineering research laboratory. In vivo, the concept of a "niche" is often used to describe the specialized microenvironment consisting of multiple cell types and signaling factors in which stem cells reside. This highly controlled niche consists of soluble cytokines, cell–cell contacts, and cell–extracellular matrix (ECM) interactions that regulate stem cell fate decisions by organizing the location, strength, and availability of exogenous factors (Davey and Zandstra 2004). Signaling may be of autocrine or paracrine nature, and stem cell position is highly localized to certain areas of the tissue. Thus, the stem cell niche may be described as a fixed-location-dependent signaling niche where positional information regulating cellular processes is provided by surrounding support cells (Davey and Zandstra 2004).

More recently, stem cell bioengineering has been concerned with the use of microscale technologies to engineer the stem cell niche. Niche engineering may be used as a technical tool for controlling stem cell fate. Applying niche engineering as a system to culture stem cells allows for tight regulation over various niche parameters, including soluble cytokines, ECM, cell–cell contacts, and niche-support cells, thus reducing the inherent heterogeneity in the culture system (Peerani 2008). Furthermore, applying these microscale technologies to stem cell culture allows molecular cues to be provided with the precision and spatial resolution that mimics that found in vivo (Peerani 2008). This sequence of laboratory sessions incorporates one of these microtechnologies: stem cell micropatterning.

Micropatterning stem cell cultures can regulate typically uncontrolled ESC culture parameters such as colony size, distance between colonies, ECM substrate, and cell–cell interactions. This technique may be considered a means to controlling niche size and spatial arrangement. Soft lithography, the micropatterning procedure used in this laboratory, involves casting an elastomeric prepolymer such as poly(dimethylsiloxane) (PDMS) onto a master silicon wafer that has been patterned with a photoresist (Figure 15.1; Appendix 5) (Chen et al. 1998; Folch and Toner 1998; Folch et al. 1999; Hwang et al. 2009). Because PDMS replicas of these wafers are biocompatible, they can be inked with an ECM solution and stamped onto a tissue culture-treated surface for use in cell culture. Cells are seeded onto the culture surface and allowed to adhere to the patterned regions.

Recently, it has been shown that use of micropatterning to control mESC colony size can be used to regulate activation of the Janus kinase–signal transducer and activator of transcription (Jak-Stat) pathway (Peerani et al. 2009). The Jak-Stat pathway is active during embryonic stem cell renewal and signaling is initiated by the interleukin-6 (IL-6) family of cytokines, including leukemia inhibitory factor (LIF), which is typically required for the maintenance of mESCs in vitro (Williams et al. 1988) (Figure 15.2).

Receptor-ligand binding, or complex formation, results in phosphorylation of the tyrosine-705 residue of STAT3 (pSTAT3) by receptor-associated Janus kinases (Jaks), which is followed by pSTAT3 translocation to the nucleus (Zhong, Wen, and Darnell 1994). At the nucleus, direct transcriptional targets of pSTAT3 include members of the Jak-Stat pathway (gp130, STAT3, suppressor of cytokine signaling 3 [Socs3], and LIF receptor [LIFR]) (Davey et al. 2007). The level of phosphorylated STAT3 (pSTAT3) can therefore be used as an indicator of endogenous signaling activation. Ultimately, nuclear levels of pSTAT3 in mESCs can be modulated in a predictive manner by altering colony diameter, the distance between colonies, and/or the degree of cell clustering (Peerani et al. 2009).

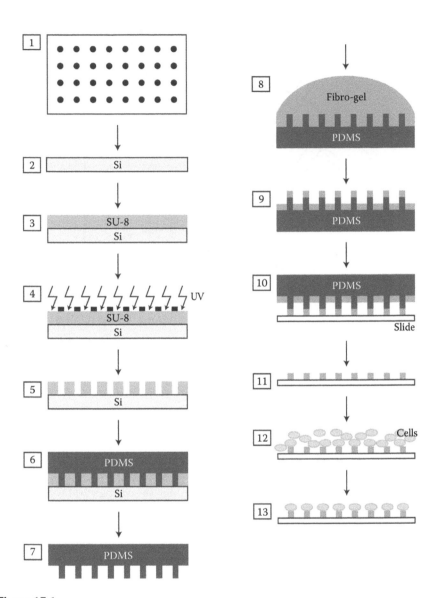

Figure 15.1
Overview of PDMS stamp fabrication for culture use. (1) A micropattern photomask is designed using CAD software and printed on a transparency. (2) A polished silicon wafer is cleaned and (3) SU-8 photoresist is spin-coated onto the surface. (4) UV light cross links exposed wafer surface areas not covered by the photomask. (5) Nonexposed regions are dissolved in SU-8 developer. (6) PDMS prepolymer is cured onto the template mold and (7) the resulting PDMS stamp is released from the mold. (8) The stamp is inked with ECM (fibronectin/gelatin) solution and (9) excess solution is removed. (10) The stamp is used to create ECM patterns on a tissue-culture-treated slide. (11) The slide is passivated in Pluronic to prevent cell attachment to non-ECM-coated regions. (12) mESCs are seeded onto the patterned surface (13) and nonattached cells are washed away.

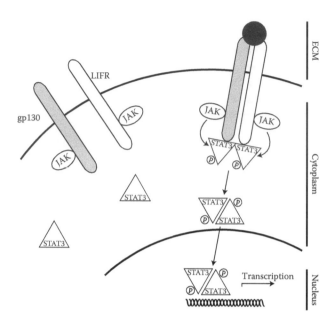

Figure 15.2
Overview of Jak-STAT3 intracellular signaling. Extracellular LIF (dark circle) binds to its receptor (LIFR) and gp130, causing receptor-associated Jak (ovals) to phosphorylate STAT3 (triangles). Phosphorylated STAT3 (triangles with circular "p") translocates to the nucleus to initiate gene transcription and promote cell survival/maintenance.

Cells probe their microenvironment and communicate with other cells through autocrine and paracrine signaling. The laboratory protocol described in this chapter uses a stochastic model that predicts the fraction of autocrine and paracrine trajectories captured by a single cell and the complex number (ligand-bound receptor) distribution among colonies in cell culture assays (Figure 15.3).

The original model (Batsilas, Berezhkovskii, and Shvartsman 2003) calculated a general solution to ligand lifetime and spatial trapping distribution. This model assumed infinite medium height, two-dimensional cell distribution, and constant and uniform distribution of ligand secretion and receptor expression. The model states that the probability density function (p) for the coordinate of a diffusion ligand at the cell surface satisfies the following:

$$D \frac{\partial p(x,y,z,t)}{\partial z}\bigg|_{z=0} = \kappa p(x,y,z=0,t) \tag{15.1}$$

where the rate constant, κ, refers to the single cell trapping efficiency and is equal to

$$\kappa = \frac{k_{on} R_t}{\pi r_{cell}^2 N_a} \tag{15.2}$$

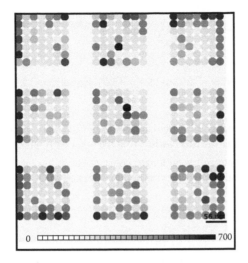

Figure 15.3
A grid pattern of cells with 10 mm radius provided by the simulation model. The grayscale lookup table indicates the scale from none (0) to high (700) for ligand/receptor complex number per cell. The model predicts the fraction of autocrine and paracrine signaling trajectories captured by a single cell and the complex number distribution among colonies in cell culture assays.

where
k_{on} is the ligand-receptor binding rate constant
R_t is the total number of receptors per cell
r_{cell} is the radius of the cell
N_a is Avogadro's number

From this calculation, equations for the autocrine and paracrine capture probabilities can be found:

$$\text{Autocrine: } \kappa = \frac{k_{on}R_t}{\pi r_{cell}^2 N_a} \tag{15.3}$$

$$\text{Paracrine: } p(r) = \frac{2\kappa_{eff}}{\pi D} \int_0^\infty \frac{x^2}{\left(\kappa_{eff} r \big/ D\right)^2 + x^2} K_0(x)\, dx \tag{15.4}$$

where
$D_a = \kappa r_{cell}/D$ is a dimensionless number called the Damkohler number
$K_o(x)$ is the modified 0th order Bessel function of the second kind
v is the internalization ratio and is equal to $k_e/(k_e + k_{off})$

κ_{eff} is the effective single-cell trapping efficiency for paracrine trajectories and is equal to

$$\kappa_{eff} = \frac{\kappa\sigma}{1+\pi D_a/4} \text{ where } \sigma = \frac{(\# cells)r_{cell}^2 \pi}{A} \tag{15.5}$$

In the extended model (Peerani et al. 2009), Equations 15.1–15.5 were altered to account for the following:

- Complex number per cell is calculated for each cell by summing the autocrine trajectories with the paracrine trajectories from the other cells on the surface.
- Receptor number per cell is no longer constant but follows a Gaussian distribution (a random receptor number from within a user-defined range is given to each cell upon model initialization).
- Complex degradation is included.

The extended model assumes that distances between cells can be divided into 1 μm increments and that complex degradation rate is constant with respect to time and independent of the number of complexes. Complex number for cell i ($(C_n)_i$) is calculated by summing the autocrine trajectories (P^i_{au}) with the paracrine trajectories from other cells on the surface (P^i_{para}). This sum is multiplied by the ligand secretion rate (v_l) minus the degradation rate and simulation time (t). All modified equations are presented next:

$$(C_n)_i = (v_i - k_{deg})(P^i_{au} + P^i_{para})t \tag{15.6}$$

$$P^i_{au} = \frac{vD^i_a}{vD^i_a + 4/\pi} \tag{15.7}$$

$$P^i_{au} = \frac{vD^i_a}{vD^i_a + 4/\pi} \tag{15.8}$$

$$p(r_{ij}) = \frac{2\kappa^i_{eff}}{\pi D} \int_0^{\infty} \frac{x^2}{(\kappa^i_{eff}r_{ij}/D)^2 + x^2} K_0(x)dx \tag{15.9}$$

This model was developed by Peter Zandstra's laboratory team at the University of Toronto and is an extension of another model developed by Stanislav Y. Shvartsman at Princeton University (Peerani et al. 2009; Batsilas, Berezhkovskii, and Shvartsman 2003). The model applies to the gp130-Jak-Stat signaling pathway and the recommended parameters for simulation were chosen based upon previous work done on this signaling pathway or similar systems (Table 15.1).

TABLE 15.1
Accepted Simulation Parameters

Parameter	Description	Value	Unit
R_t	Total receptors per cell	300–00	#
R_{cell}	Radius of a cell	10	μm
D	Diffusivity of LIF (IL-6)	2.7×10^{-7}	cm^2/s
k_{on}	Association rate constant	0.2×10^9	$M^{-1} min^{-1}$
k_{off}	Dissociation rate constant	0.0011	min^{-1}
k_e	Endocytosis rate constant	0.0099	min^{-1}
k_{deg}	Degradation rate of complexes	0.2	min^{-1}
v_1	Ligand secretion rate	0.831	#/min
Time	Simulation time	24	h

15.2 Learning Objectives

The objectives of this experiment are to

- Gain an understanding of the complementary nature of in silico and in vitro experimental approaches
- Gain a deeper understanding of the nature of autocrine and paracrine signaling
- Engage in the design of a novel experiment using newly gained knowledge from the literature
- Gain experience with soft lithography, PDMS fabrication, micropatterning, stem cell culture, immunostaining, and fluorescence microscopy
- Develop a basic understanding of stem cell biology

15.3 Overview of Experiment

This laboratory combines in silico and in vitro techniques to investigate how stem cell niche size controls endogenous signaling thresholds in mouse embryonic stem cells (mESCs). Specifically, a mathematical model of autocrine and paracrine signaling is used in combination with a stem cell micropatterning technique to investigate how spatial control over stem cell arrangement modulates paracrine signaling in the Jak-Stat pathway.

The entire laboratory consists of seven sessions. The first laboratory session serves as an introduction to the model. Considerable student preparation is required prior to session 2, where individual student experiments and pattern templates are designed. Sessions 3–7 involve other techniques to fabricate, execute, and confirm a novel experiment. Refer to Appendix 5 for an overview of the fabrication process. *Note: Due to the nature of the required protocols, sessions 5–7 should be held during a consecutive 3-day period.*

The recommended laboratory schedule is as follows:

Session 1: directed simulation (modeling software)

Session 2: creation of computer-aided design (CAD) patterns and definition of experimental plan

Session 3: Master fabrication

Session 4: PDMS stamp fabrication

Session 5: Micropatterning of mESCs (overnight)

Session 6: Immunofluorescent labeling of pSTAT3 as an indicator of Jak-Stat pathway activation (overnight incubation)

Session 7: Completion of pSTAT3 immunostaining and pattern assessment

15.4 Safety Notes

Sessions 3 and 4: If masters and PDMS stamps are fabricated in a cleanroom facility, specific safety training will be required in order to work within the facility. Generally, the full body should be covered by a "bunny suit" (cleanroom coverall) to work in such an environment. This not only protects the wearer from minor spills and splashes but also helps keep the room clean. Boot covers should be worn over closed-toe shoes, and a hair net/cap and safety goggles must also be worn. *If masters and stamps are fabricated in a general lab environment, a lab coat, gloves, and goggles must be worn (refer to Appendix 5).* Follow all chemical MSDS safety precautions. Be certain to work within a fume hood when handling SU-8 developer, curing reagents, and other solvents and handle box cutters carefully. Also familiarize yourself with proper reagent disposal.

    Session 5: Always wear gloves and a lab coat when handling stem cell preparations. Dispose of reagents appropriately. Use the N_2 gun in a well-ventilated area.

    Session 6: Consult the MSDS if uncertain about handling formaldehyde. Wear nitrile gloves, protective goggles, and a lab coat and always work in a fume hood when handling formalin. Formalin and consequent wash solutions should be disposed of as directed for chemical waste. Also use caution when handling Hoechst/DAPI solutions. These are suspected carcinogens and waste should be discarded accordingly.

15.5 Materials

15.5.1 Reagents and Disposables

- SU-8 2050 Photoresist
- Silicon wafers (single side polished; 3 in × 0.5 mm thickness)
- Acetate transparencies for laser printer
- Petri dishes (>15 cm; soda lime silica glass)
- SU-8 Developer fluid
- Isopropyl alcohol

- 15 cm petri dishes (plastic)
- Sylgard®184 silicone elastomer kit (PDMS)
- Pluronic® F-127
- Sterile deionized H_2O (dH_2O)
- 100% Ethanol
- Nunc microscope slides (27 × 75 mm; polystyrene tissue culture treated)
- Fibronectin/gelatin ECM solution
- mESC Serum-free media
- mESC Media with serum
- Trypsin-EDTA
- mESCs (ATCC SCRC-1011™; designation R1; 1 × T25 flask)
- Trypan blue
- Chamber slides (e.g., Nunc Lab-Tek II; eight-well pack/16)
- 10% Neutral buffered formalin
- Methanol
- Block buffer: 10% normal goat serum (NGS) in phosphate-buffered saline (PBS)
- Dilution/wash buffer: 3% NGS in PBS
- Primary antibody solution: Phospho-Stat3 (Tyr705) antibody in dilution/wash buffer
- Secondary antibody solution: AlexaFluor® 488 goat antirabbit antibody in dilution/wash buffer
- Normal rabbit IgG (NRIgG; immunostaining control)
- Hoechst 33342 (or DAPI)

15.5.2 Equipment and Supplies

- Modeling software (available from http://www.crcpress.com/product/isbn/9781439878934)
- CAD software
- Agitator (e.g., "belly dancer" orbital shaker)
- Sterile metal forceps or large tweezers
- Thirsties fab wipes
- Chemat precision spin-coater
- Chemat UV curer
- Chemat compact hotplate, programmable
- Box cutter
- N_2 gun (Entegris)
- Silicone gasket isolators (e.g., Grace Bio Labs #664301 or #665304)
- Humidifier (e.g., Sunbeam model 697)
- Plexiglas humidity chamber

- Microscope equipped for fluorescence and digital imaging (filter for viewing AlexaFluor 488 [EX: 488 nm, EM: 519 nm] and Hoechst 33342 or DAPI [EX: 350 nm, EM: 461 nm])

15.6 Recipes

5% (w/v) Pluronic F-127. Mix 5 g of Pluronic F-127 in 100 mL autoclaved dH_2O. Filter-sterilize using a bottle top filter.

Serum-free seeding media. Add Dulbecco's modified Eagle's medium (DMEM) supplemented with 15% KNOCKOUT™ serum replacement, 50 mg penicillin–streptomycin (P/S), 2 mM l-glutamine, 0.1 mM 2-mercaptoethanol, and 500 pM leukemia inhibitory factor (LIF); sterile-filter prior to use.

Media with serum. Add DMEM supplemented with 15% fetal bovine serum (FBS), 50 mg P/S, 2 mM l-glutamine, 0.1 mM 2-mercaptoethanol, and 500 pM LIF; sterile-filter prior to use.

Fibronectin/gelatin ECM solution. Prepare 50 mg/mL gelatin (from bovine skin) solution in dH_2O and autoclave; combine 1 mL of 0.1% fibronectin (from bovine plasma) with 39 mL of gelatin solution.

Block buffer. Mix 1.25 mL of NGS in 23.75 mL PBS; while stirring, add 75 µL Triton X-100.

Dilution/wash buffer. Mix 1.2 mL of NGS in 38.8 mL PBS; while stirring, add 120 µL of Triton X-100.

Primary antibody solution. Dilute phosphoStat3 (Tyr-705) primary antibody 1:100 in antibody dilution buffer (i.e., 5 µL antibody + 495 µL of buffer); keep on ice and discard unused portion of aliquot.

Control antibody solution. Dilute normal rabbit IgG 1:400 in antibody dilution buffer (i.e., 1.25 µL NRIgG + 487.5 µL of buffer); keep on ice and discard unused portion of aliquot.

Secondary antibody solution. Dilute AlexaFluor 488 goat antirabbit antibody 1:2000 in antibody dilution buffer; wrap aliquot in aluminum foil and keep on ice; discard unused portion of aliquot.

Hoechst 33342 solution. Dilute 10 mg/mL Hoechst stock 1:5000 in PBS; wrap aliquot in foil and keep on ice; discard unused portion of aliquot.

DAPI (alternative to Hoechst). Add 2 mL of dH_2O to the contents of one vial (creates 5 mg/mL stock solution); to prepare the working solution, dilute stock to 300 nM in PBS; keep aliquot wrapped in foil and store at 4°C for up to 6 months.

15.7 Methods

15.7.1 Session 1: Directed Model Simulation

This laboratory session allows you to investigate and become familiar with the mathematical model described in the background section. By the end of this session, you should be familiar enough with the model to apply it to your own experimental design. It is strongly suggested that you refer to the referenced literature describing

the model **before** coming to the lab. The modeling software is available at http://
www.crcpress.com/product/isbn/9781439878934. *All coordinate files referred to
may be found in the "Testfiles" folder accompanying the model.* Specific questions
have been included to guide you through the software.

15.7.1.1 Stochastic Model of Autocrine and Paracrine Signaling Users Guide

- Overview and requirements. The stochastic model of autocrine and paracrine signaling was written in the Python computing language. Your instructor has installed the
  following packages on the lab computers to run the model: Python 2.5.4, Scipy 0.9.0.
  Numpy 1.6.1, Pmw 1.3.2, and Matplotlib 1.0.1. Although the program may run under
  more recent versions of Python, code compatibility with versions more recent than
  2.5.4 has not been extensively tested. The graphical user interface (Figure 15.4) can be
  used by running App.py in the IDLE integrated development environment.

- **Loading a coordinate file.** To load a coordinate file, select "Open Coord" at the top
  left of the screen (Figure 15.4). You may load any set of coordinates with a .txt or
  .py format. Coordinate files must begin with two lines of comments (beginning with
  "#") followed by the number of cells. For an example, refer to the "Testfiles" folder of
  coordinates. Once a coordinate file is opened, the program will automatically compute
  the necessary probabilities and statistics; thus, there is no need to select "Compute."
  Cell arrangements may be viewed in different modes and in different color scaling
  (Table 15.2 provides descriptions).

- **Changing parameters.** All parameters under "User Set Parameters" may be changed.
  Simply type in the desired parameter and select "Update" at the top of the screen.
  "Update" will automatically update all parameters and recalculate all probabilities and

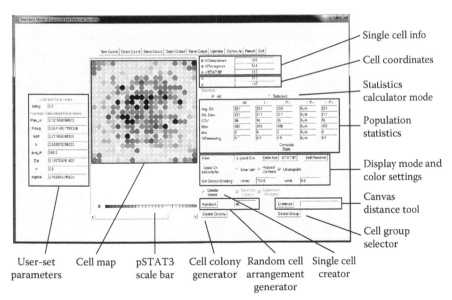

Single cell info

Cell coordinates

Statistics
calculator mode

Population
statistics

Display mode and
color settings

Canvas
distance tool

Cell group
selector

User-set   Cell map   pSTAT3   Cell colony   Random cell   Single cell
parameters   scale bar   generator   arrangement   creator
                                                    generator

Figure 15.4
Annotated graphical users interface.

TABLE 15.2
Stochastic Model Software Button Descriptions

Button	Description
New Coord	Clears existing cell coordinates in preparation for a new set of coordinates
Open Coord	Allows selection of a coordinate set in .txt or .py format
Save Coord	Saves current coordinates, whether generated within canvas or preloaded. Appropriate file type must be manually added (.txt or .py)
Open Output	Opens preexisting output files (.txt or .py); will display statistics and load cell arrangement
Save Output	Saves the computed population statistics and single cell information (coordinates, Cn, pSTAT3, self-renewal) in user-specified file type
Update	Updates altered parameters
Compute	Computes cell population and single statistics
Reset	Resets all parameters to accepted values
Quit	Quits simulator
Statistics	To select whether to display statistics from entire population (All) or for a selected group
Ligand Dist.	Display based on the calculated ligand distribution
Definition	Displays the definition of all cell coordinates with a uniform color distribution
STAT3P	Displays based on pSTAT3 scale bar and single-cell pSTAT3 levels
Self-Renewal	Displays which cells are likely to self-renew based on a threshold level of pSTAT3 per cell
Scale Intensity	Sets intensity of color for scale bar
Color Scaling	Sets color display mode
Create Mode	Creates single cells with optional settings for ligand secretion and receptor expression
Random	Generates a random nonoverlapping arrangement of a user-specified number of cells
Distance	Calculates the distance in microns of a user-created line on the canvas
Create Colony	Creates a tightly packed colony of cells within a user-defined rectangular region
Select Group	Highlights a group of user-selected cells for further statistical calculation with the statistics function "Select Group" option

statistics. Parameters may be reset to the original default values by selecting "Reset" at the top of screen. Probabilities and statistics will automatically be recalculated.

- **Creating a colony.** The "Create Colony" button at the bottom right of the screen may be used to create rectangular colonies anywhere on the canvas. Simply clear the current colony by clicking on "New Coord" (if a fresh coordinate file is desired), select "Create Colony," and create rectangles on the canvas using the cursor. The program automatically recalculates all probabilities and statistics after each colony has been drawn.

- **Creating a random arrangement.** The "Random" button at the bottom right of the screen will create a random nonoverlapping cell arrangement with the number of cells indicated in the text box located to the right of the button. To change the number of cells, type in the desired number and select "Update." To initiate generation of the cell arrangement, select the button and subsequently use the cursor to click anywhere on the canvas. Select the "Compute" button to calculate all probabilities and statistics.

- **Using single-cell placement.** Select "Create Mode" to create single cells on the canvas using the cursor. Simply click anywhere on the canvas to create a cell. Cells may be created with or without receptors for ligands and with or without the potential to secrete ligands. "Compute" must be selected subsequent to creation of the desired cell arrangement to calculate probabilities and statistics.

- **Calculating canvas distances.** Distances on the canvas may be calculated by selecting "Distance" at the bottom right of the screen and drawing a line anywhere on the canvas using the cursor. The distance in microns (μm) will subsequently be displayed in the text box to the right of the "Distance" button.

- **Statistics.** Unless otherwise specified, probabilities and statistics are calculated on a population basis. Single cells may be selected to display single cell coordinates, receptor, and complex numbers. These will be displayed in the top right of the screen. To calculate statistics for a group of cells, select the "Select Group" button at the bottom right of the screen, select a group using the cursor, select the "Selected" option under statistics, and press the "Compute" button located under the statistics display.

- **Saving outputs.** Select "Save Output" at the top of the screen to save the current coordinates and corresponding probabilities and statistics. The format (.py or .txt) must be manually typed following the desired file name.

- **Opening outputs.** To open a past output, select "Open Output" at the top of the screen. The cell coordinates will be loaded and probabilities and statistics calculated.

15.7.1.2 Investigate Model Parameters

The dependency of the model on its parameters will be examined initially. To do this, the cell pattern is kept constant while model parameters are altered to investigate the resultant change in complex number (C_n) and endogenous STAT3 activation. Use a square, tightly packed arrangement of 400 cells (Pattern1.txt). Initiate the model using the accepted parameters (Table 15.1) and a cell surface area of 314,159 μm² (for 40% coverage). The following questions will assist your thinking as you work through the model:

1. Based on what you have read about the model, are the cells uniformly secreting ligands? Investigate the change in pSTAT3 levels with an increase/decrease in ligand secretion rate (v_1). Explain why pSTAT3 levels are highest at the center of the cell arrangement. Are the autocrine and paracrine capture probabilities dependent on this parameter (v_1)?

2. Using the model output for number 1, choose one cell at the edge of the arrangement and one cell at the center of the arrangement. With the model equations provided previously, calculate the autocrine capture probability for each cell. Comment on your findings.

3. Increase the number of cell surface receptors by increasing Rt_{max}. How does the average complex number (C_n) change? How do the single-cell pSTAT3 levels change? Why? How does altering R_t affect the single-cell trapping efficiency (κ)? Comment on the resultant effect on the autocrine and paracrine capture probabilities.

4. How are receptor numbers being assigned to cells in this model? If each cell has a different receptor number, what other parameters will be different for each cell? Which

parameters are the same for all cells? If receptor number was assumed to be constant across all cells, how would the autocrine/paracrine capture probabilities change?

5. Increase, then decrease, the area of the bioreactor (A). How do the single-cell pSTAT3 levels change? Why? For this model, is autocrine capture probability dependent upon the density of cells? In this case, to what is the change in single-cell pSTAT3 levels largely attributed?

6. Increase, then decrease, the diffusivity of the ligand (D). What happens to single-cell pSTAT3 levels? Why? Provide an explanation for your observation in terms of what is occurring at the cellular level. Comment on how the diffusivity of the ligand affects the autocrine and paracrine capture probabilities.

7. The expression for autocrine capture probability in this model represents the probability for both recapture and internalization of the ligand. Show mathematically how this expression would change if it accounted only for recapture. Explain the significance of the Damkohler number (D_a) in terms of the autocrine capture probability.

15.7.1.3 Investigate Niche Size Parameters

In this section you will explore how niche size controls endogenous STAT3 activation. The model parameters are kept constant (at the accepted values), while differing cell arrangements to the model are introduced. All cell arrangements may be found in the "Testfiles" folder.

1. Thus far, a patterned arrangement of 400 cells has been used. Random0.txt–Random5. txt are nonoverlapping coordinates for random cell arrangements ranging from 0.3 to 0.8 surface coverage. Run each of these files with the areas indicated in Table 15.3. Run Pattern1.txt with these same areas. Copy the table to your laboratory notebook and record the average complex formation number for each condition. Plot C_n versus surface coverage (σ) for the patterned and random cases and investigate the trends. Specifically, investigate how the difference in endogenous STAT3 activation between patterned and random arrangements changes with increasing cell surface coverage. At what point does patterning stop having a positive effect on single-cell pSTAT3 levels? Why? Based on what you are observing, what is the advantage of micropatterned cells?

2. In question 1 of Section 15.7.1.2, the difference in C_n between patterned and random arrangements of cells at the same surface coverage was observed. How does the *local* cell density differ between patterned and random arrangements? Is it the local

TABLE 15.3
Test Files and Associated Surface Areas

Surface Coverage (σ)	File Name (Random)	Area (μm^2)	Pattern C_n	Random C_n
0.3	Random0.txt	418,879		
0.4	Random1.txt	314,159		
0.5	Random2.txt	251,327		
0.6	Random3.txt	209,439		
0.7	Random4.txt	179,519		
0.8	Random5.txt	157,079		

TABLE 15.4
Test Files and Associated Surface Areas

File Name	Diameter (µm)	Pitch (µm)	Area (µm²)	C_n
Pattern2a.txt	100	20	360,000	
Pattern2b.txt	100	40	360,000	
Pattern2c.txt	100	60	360,000	
Pattern3a.txt	100	100	291,600	
Pattern3b.txt	120	80	291,600	
Pattern3c.txt	140	60	291,600	

microenvironment of a cell or the well's macroscopic environment that correlates with endogenous signal activation of a single cell?

3. Other than soluble ligand availability and binding, what other extrinsic factor(s) may contribute to phenotypic changes in stem cell cultures?

4. In question 3 of Section 15.7.1.2, extrinsic factors that may contribute to phenotypic changes in stem cell cultures were identified. Explain how micropatterning of stem cell cultures may affect these extrinsic variables. Comment on the advantageous nature of this approach with respect to investigating soluble ligand availability and binding.

5. As defined for this model, κ_{eff} is the single-cell trapping efficiency for paracrine trajectories. In question 3 of Section 15.7.1.2, it was determined that κ_{eff} is different for every cell due to differing receptor numbers. Will κ_{eff} change for differing cell arrangements kept at the same cell surface coverage? Explain. What implications does this have for investigating micropatterning with this model?

6. Cell arrangements Pattern2a.txt, Pattern2b.txt, and Pattern2c.txt (Table 15.4) are patterned arrangements of cells comprising nine colonies with constant diameter and increasing pitch (separation). Area should be held constant at 360,000 µm². Investigate how endogenous STAT3 activation changes with increasing pitch. In increasing pitch, what is happening to the *local* cell density?

7. Cell arrangements Pattern3a.txt, Pattern3b.txt, and Pattern3c.txt (Table 15.4) are patterned arrangements of cells comprising nine colonies with increasing colony diameter. Area should be held constant at 291,600 µm². Investigate how endogenous STAT3 activation changes with increasing colony diameter. What is happening to the *local* cell density?

8. Increasing local cell density has an effect on endogenous STAT3 activation. If you were given a flask of cells at 30% cell surface coverage and asked to increase the surface coverage to 40% by adding more cells to the flask, would you expect to see an increase in endogenous activation?

15.7.2 Session 2: Experiment Pattern Design and Proposal

Taking advantage of what you have researched in the literature about mESC micropatterning in combination with the mathematical model used in session 1, propose an experiment to investigate how niche size and stem cell arrangement modulate activation of the Jak-Stat pathway. Restrict the experimental proposal to the design of one or two micropatterns and include measurement of pSTAT3 translocation to the nucleus as a measure of Jak-Stat activation. The cellular levels of pSTAT3 will be identified and quantified by immunostaining; therefore, consider the appropriate controls that should be included.

The experimental protocol should meet the following specifications:

- Be completed within the allocated time of each laboratory session
- Involve the design of a novel patterning scheme (create using CAD software of your choice)
- Focus on investigating some change in pSTAT3 level with cell arrangement
- Use relevant literature to support the hypothesis and pattern design
- Include proper controls

Using the modeling software provided, test your hypothesis prior to performing the experiment by running simulations of your pattern(s). You may also use the software to assist in your experimental design. These predictions and results should be included in your proposal.

Use CAD software of your choice to create the pattern(s) you intend to test. Prior to session 3, these patterns should be printed on transparency using a laser printer at a resolution higher than 5600 dpi. Pattern features must remain within the range of 200–800 μm and fit within a 20 mm circular silicone gasket. Be sure that the pattern features are **solid black** and draw a box around each pattern with text describing the patterns.

The written proposal should include the following:

- **Background.** Discuss the principles and/or theories that will form the basis of the hypothesis. This section serves to justify your hypothesis.
- **Hypothesis.** Outline a clear and testable hypothesis for the experiment.
- **Experimental plan.** Briefly outline the experimental approach that will be used to test the hypothesis. Include a description and diagram of the proposed pattern. Be sure to include proper controls.
- **Expected results.** Based on what you have read and learned, describe what you believe will be the outcome of your experiment. Discuss expected quantitative results (e.g., pattern 1 will increase complex formation to a greater degree than pattern 2). Include graphs or charts if and where appropriate.

15.7.3 Session 3: Fabricate Master

During this laboratory session, photomasks of student patterns will be used to create device "masters" that will be used in session 4 to fabricate PDMS stamps by soft lithography. The TA or lab instructor will ensure that CAD patterns are printed to acetate transparencies using a high-resolution laser printer and are available at this session. *Note: The following describes master creation in a cleanroom facility. Refer to Figure 15.1 for overview.*

1. Preheat two digital hotplates to 65°C and 95°C, *respectively*. These are used to heat the silicon wafer gradually.

2. Place a silicon wafer on the 65°C hotplate for 1 min. Use metal forceps to transfer the silicon wafer subsequently to the 95°C hotplate for 1 min. Transfer the wafer to a clean petri dish to cool (glass or plastic). *It is recommended that the side chosen to handle the silicon wafer is kept constant throughout the procedure.*

3. Slowly pour enough SU-8 2050 to cover half of the wafer. Begin by pouring slightly off-center of the wafer and moving in one direction to just past center. *This minimizes bubbles by avoiding SU-8 buildup on top of itself and will ensure that the SU-8 is poured onto the center of the wafer.*

4. Aluminum foil should cover the spin coater and be clean without any holes. Place the wafer onto the spin coater and center it.

5. Run the spin coater* as follows:

   Step 0: leave blank

   Step 1: 10 s dwell (at 500 rpm) with a 5 s ramp

   Step 2: 30 s dwell (at 1500 rpm) with a 5 s ramp

   Step 3: 0 s dwell (0 rpm) with a 5 s ramp

6. Carefully remove the wafer from the spin coater and transfer to the 65°C hotplate for 5 min, followed by 95°C for 25–30 min. Allow the wafer to cool for 5–10 min.

7. In preparation for UV exposure, turn on the lamp and allow it to heat up for 5 min.

8. Transfer the cooled wafer to the UV stand and place the photomask over it. Expose the wafer to UV light for 8.1 s.

9. Transfer the exposed wafer to the 65°C hotplate for 5 min, followed by the 95°C hotplate for 10 min. Allow to cool for 5–10 min.

10. Rinse a glass petri dish with SU-8 developer fluid: fill the dish with enough fresh SU-8 developer fluid just to cover the wafer. Place the wafer carefully into the dish and gently agitate (at approximately speed level 3) for not more than 10 min. Work in the fume hood when handling the SU-8 developer fluid.

11. Use forceps to lift the wafer carefully out of the developer fluid. While holding the wafer over the glass dish, rinse with isopropyl alcohol from a squeeze bottle for ~10 s. *The formation of a white film at this stage indicates underdevelopment. Submerse the wafer in the developer fluid once more to remove the white film and repeat the rinse.* If no white film is present, rinse with SU-8 developer fluid from a squeeze bottle.

12. Place the clean wafer on a clean fab wipe and allow to air dry for 5 min. Dry the wafer completely with nitrogen gas and store in a clean 15 cm plastic petri dish (with lid).

---

* Settings will depend on the specific spin coater. Confirm with facility staff. Target thickness is 70–75 μm.

15.7.4 Session 4: Fabricate PDMS Stamp

1. Place the wafer in a safe place at a PDMS-designated workbench.

2. The PDMS mixture is a two-part silicone elastomer. Use a scale and glass beaker to weigh out a 10:1 ratio of base to curing agent. Approximately 60 g of PDMS mixture is required per stamp. Stir the mixture vigorously for 5 min.

3. Pour PDMS mixture slowly over the wafer until a height of 3–4 mm is achieved. Ensure that the wafer is centered in the petri dish and that it is fully covered by PDMS.

4. Place the petri dish into the vacuum chamber at –20 mm Hg pressure for 20–25 min. *This is required to remove bubbles from the PDMS mixture.*

5. Once all bubbles have been removed, cure the PDMS in a curing oven at 80°C for 1 h.

6. The PDMS is now ready to be made into a stamp. Remove from the oven and cut away excess PDMS as follows:

    a. Use a box cutter to cut a pentagon shape around the wafer. Ensure that the cuts traverse the entire depth of the PDMS.

    b. Carefully work your way around the pentagon to lift the wafer (with PDMS attached) out of the petri dish.

    c. Place the wafer on a clean surface of the bench with the PDMS side down. Trace around the wafer with a blade to remove the excess PDMS.

    d. Carefully peel away the thin layer of PDMS that has cured to the backside of the wafer. *This will make it easier to detach the wafer from the PDMS.*

    e. Slowly detach the PDMS from the wafer and place the wafer back into the petri dish. Avoid touching the patterned surface of the PDMS to minimize residual fingerprints.

7. Cut out stamps from the PDMS and place into a small petri dish.

8. Fill the dish with 70% ethanol (cover the stamps) and let stand overnight to sterilize.

15.7.5 Session 5: Microcontact Printing and Stem Cell Plating

In this laboratory session, the PDMS stamps created in session 4 are used to pattern mESCs onto tissue culture-treated slides. *Note: Remember to stamp the appropriate number of regions for use as immunostaining controls.*

1. UV-sterilize the silicone gaskets for 10 min on each side. Remember to use a sufficient number to create enough patterns to include the controls you have chosen.

2. Turn on the humidifier in the humidifying chamber. The chamber should reach a relative humidity of 55%–70%.

3. Prepare the biological safety cabinet (BSC) for use by wiping down with 70% ethanol and arranging necessary reagents and disposables.

4. In the BSC, transfer the stamps to a sterile petri dish and allow to air dry. Use sterile forceps to turn the stamps and allow both sides to dry fully.

5. Once dry, transfer 1 mL of fibronectin/gelatin solution onto the patterned side of the stamp. Gently pipette up and down to spread evenly. Let stand in the BSC for 1 h at room temperature (RT) in a covered petri dish.

6. After 1 h, pour excess fibronectin/gelatin into another petri dish. Hold the stamp over the waste dish and use a micropipette to rinse with dH_2O. Use a N_2 gun to dry the stamp until there are no water droplets remaining on the surface of the stamp. Proceed to the next step *immediately* as allowing the stamp to overdry (i.e., leaving for >1 min) will result in poor transfer and protein denaturation.

7. Stamp your pattern onto a tissue culture-treated slide while working within the humidifying chamber. Carefully lower the stamp onto the slide in one movement. *Try not to move the stamp once it touches the slide as this will cause the pattern to smear.*

8. Tap the stamp **lightly** before gently placing a glass slide over it, followed by a small weight (e.g., small glass bottle or beaker). This ensures that uniform pressure is applied between the stamp and the tissue culture slide. Be gentle as the stamp is very shallow. Let stand for 8–10 min.

9. Remove the weight and carefully lift the top glass slide. The stamp should stick to the top glass slide.

10. Place a silicone gasket around your stamped pattern and press firmly to ensure a tight seal. Any leakage will result in cell culture failure.

11. Use a micropipette to add sufficient Pluronic to cover the pattern. Let stand for 1 h at 4°C.

12. Prepare the mESCs for seeding during this 1 h incubation period:

    a. Remove the cells from the incubator.

    b. View the cells under the microscope. Note the cell morphology and extent of confluence.

    c. Trypsinize the cells (refer to trypsinization protocol in Appendix 1; however, *incubate the cells with trypsin for only 2 min*); rinse once in 4 mL media.

    d. Resuspend the cells in 2–3 mL of serum-free media.

    e. Count the cells using a hemacytometer (refer to hemacytometer protocol in Appendix 2).

    f. Dilute the suspension. The final concentration depends upon the surface coverage of your pattern. A range of $1–5 \times 10^5$ cells/gasket is sufficient for one 20 mm silicone gasket. (A 750 µL volume of cell suspension is required to fill one 20 mm gasket; therefore, calculate cell volume appropriately. Consider the number of gaskets including test and control samples.)

13. Pipette 750 µL of cell suspension into each gasket and incubate at 37°C in a covered petri dish overnight.

15.7.6 Session 6: Label pSTAT3 as an Indicator of Jak-Stat Pathway Activation

Immunofluorescence labeling is used to identify variations in pSTAT3 intensity levels and cellular localization within differentially micropatterned cultures. The level of fluorescence intensity directly reflects the amount of pSTAT3 per pattern

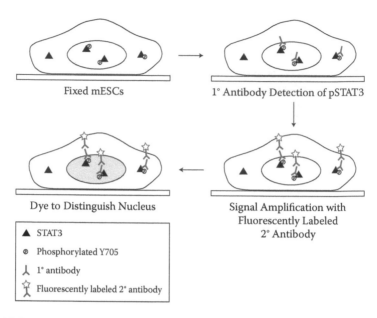

Fixed mESCs   1° Antibody Detection of pSTAT3

Dye to Distinguish Nucleus   Signal Amplification with Fluorescently Labeled 2° Antibody

▲ STAT3

⊚ Phosphorylated Y705

⅄ 1° antibody

☆ Fluorescently labeled 2° antibody

Figure 15.5
Overview of pSTAT3 fluorescent immunodetection. The primary antibody specifically recognizes the phosphorylated Tyr-705 residue of STAT3. A species-specific fluorescently labeled secondary antibody recognizes the primary antibody and amplifies the detection signal. Visualization of a nuclear dye enables quantification of cell number per colony.

and is therefore an indicator of the level of Jak-Stat pathway activation. The protocol is based upon antibody recognition of the phosphorylated Tyr-705 residue of STAT3 and consequent amplification of primary antibody signal using a fluorescently labeled secondary antibody (Figure 15.5). *Note: Aliquots of serum-free media and formalin should be prewarmed in a 37°C water bath prior to the lab session. Antibody dilution solutions should also be prepared and stored on ice immediately before the lab session. It is optimal to perform aspiration steps at a lab bench with vacuum aspiration.*

1. Obtain slides from the 37°C incubator and transfer to the lab bench.
2. Visualize the cell culture using the transmitted microscope. Acquire several images of each sample to determine the number of adherent cells prior to fixation. Save these image files.
3. *Carefully* aspirate culture media from each sample-containing gasket using a P1000 pipette. *Note: It is very easy to wash cells away if pipetting is too aggressive. Exchange wash buffers slowly.*

    Wash each sample gasket three times with prewarmed serum-free media to remove nonadherent cells. Do not pipette directly onto the cell surface. Discard wash to the appropriate waste container for eventual decontamination with bleach. Before removing the last wash, samples should be revisualized on the transmitted light microscope to determine if there is any change in adherent cell number postwash. Representative images should be acquired and compared to images taken prewash.

4. Transfer samples to a fume hood. *Note: It is important from this step forward that samples remain hydrated. Loss of sample hydration will interfere with antibody–antigen interactions.*

5. Aspirate the final wash in the fume hood and add 750 μL of 10% neutral buffered formalin solution to each gasket. Incubate for 15 min at RT. If samples are left longer than 15 min, excessive cross-linking of proteins may occur, which can result in reduced antibody detection.

6. Aspirate the formalin solution from the gaskets and dispose of in a proper waste container.

7. Wash away traces of formalin buffer by adding 750 μL PBS/gasket (leave 2 min/wash at RT). Repeat two more times to wash fully and discard wash buffer appropriately.

8. Add 750 μL methanol (100%) per gasket and incubate for 2 min at RT.

9. Aspirate the methanol quickly and dispose in a proper waste container. Immediately add 750 μL PBS buffer/gasket. Wash one gasket at a time as methanol evaporates very quickly.

10. Wash three times with 750 μL PBS/gasket (see step 7). Samples may be transferred to a regular lab bench to continue the protocol.

11. Add 750 μL block solution (10% NGS/PBS) to each gasket and incubate for 30 min at RT. *This step reduces nonspecific antibody binding.*

12. Aspirate the block solution. Add 145 μL/gasket diluted primary antibody solution to each test sample. Similarly, add 145 μL control NRIgG solution to the control sample gasket. Slides must be kept in a humidified chamber (i.e., return slides to the original petri dish in which they were stored; place folded lab tissues to the sides of the dish and soak with dH$_2$O from a squeeze bottle; place lid on the dish). Incubate samples at 4°C overnight. *Troubleshooting may be required to determine optimal immunodetection conditions.*

15.7.7 Session 7: Complete pSTAT3 Immunostaining and Pattern Assessment

1. Remove samples from overnight storage to the lab bench.

2. Aspirate buffer from each gasket. Wash gaskets three times with 750 μL/gasket wash buffer (5 min/wash at RT).

3. Add 145 μL/gasket secondary antibody solution and incubate for 45 min at RT. Keep the dish wrapped in aluminum foil under humidified conditions to protect from light.

4. Aspirate buffer from each gasket. Wash gaskets three times with 750 μL/gasket wash buffer (5 min/wash at RT).

5. Add 145 μL/gasket diluted nuclear stain (Hoechst or DAPI). Incubate Hoechst solution for 15 min at RT (or DAPI solution for 5 min at RT). Cover with aluminum foil to protect from light.

6. Aspirate the nuclear stain solution and dispose according to appropriate waste procedures. Wash each gasket three times with 750 μL PBS/gasket.

7. After the final wash is aspirated, use forceps to remove each gasket and mount a glass coverslip over each sample using Fluoromount™ mounting media (per manufacturer's recommendations). Samples may be protected from light and stored at 4°C if observation will occur during another session.

Samples should be observed using a fluorescent microscope acquisition system equipped with filters to excite the pSTAT3-associated fluorescence maximally (EX: 488 nm, EM: 519 nm) and nuclear-associated (EX: 350 nm, EM: 461 nm) signals.

It is recommended to acquire images for a minimum of five fields of view per pattern using a high-magnification objective lens. Subsequently select a low-magnification objective lens and capture images revealing a larger field of each pattern. *Note: It is extremely important to keep the exposure time the same for all images acquired for each fluorophore in order to compare fluorescence intensity levels directly. Phase contrast images should also be acquired for each field of view to assess overall cell culture.*

Imaging software can be used to analyze pSTAT3-associated intensity values for comparison between samples. ImageJ is Java-based image analysis software offered by the National Institutes of Health that can be downloaded for free. Consult the associated documentation for relevant user instructions.

15.8 Data Processing

1. Create a figure showing total cell number before and after washing the cell cultures (see session 6, steps 2 and 3). Use appropriate scale bars and labels.

2. Use appropriate labels and scale bars to create figures showing representative pSTAT3-associated fluorescence. Consider using a look-up table for figures of fields of view at low magnification. These figures should include images of 488-associated fluorescence overlaid to the corresponding images of nuclear stain and phase contrast.

3. Graphically demonstrate the distribution of pSTAT3-associated fluorescence intensity levels for the analyzed pattern(s).

15.9 Prelab Questions

1. Consider other mechanisms by which cell signaling might be regulated in this type of cell culture to maintain mESC pluripotency.

2. Why are samples incubated with formalin—and, consequently, methanol—prior to immunostaining?

3. List two immunostaining controls and describe why these should be included in the experimental protocol.

15.10 Postlab Questions

1. How can you determine if microcontact printing was successful before completing cell culture and immunofluorescent staining?

2. Compare the distribution of pSTAT3 levels per pattern identified by stimulation to the distribution of pSTAT3 levels per pattern obtained in the in vitro experiment. How were these distributions similar and how they were different?

3. Why does colony size impact STAT3 activation?

4. What role do you think colony spacing plays?

5. How do you think other shapes may behave? Specifically, what other parameters may be controlled by micropatterning cells?

6. How is STAT3 linked to stem cell self-renewal and differentiation in mouse ESCs?

7. Can you predict what role convection would have on the patterned colonies? In what equation would convection need to be integrated?

References

Batsilas, L., A. M. Berezhkovskii, and S. Y. Shvartsman. 2003. Stochastic model of autocrine and paracrine signals in cell culture assays. *Biophysics Journal* 85 (6): 3659–3665.

Chen, C. S., M. Mrksich, S. Huang, G. M. Whitesides, and D. E. Ingber. 1998. Micropatterned surfaces for control of cell shape, position, and function. *Biotechnology Progress* 14 (3): 356–363.

Davey, R. E., K. Onishi, A. Mahdavi, and P. W. Zandstra. 2007. LIF-mediated control of embryonic stem cell self-renewal emerges due to an autoregulatory loop. *FASEB Journal* 21 (9): 2020–2032.

Davey, R. E., and P. W. Zandstra. 2004. Signal processing underlying extrinsic control of stem cell fate. *Current Opinion in Hematology* 11 (2): 95–101.

Evans, M. J., and M. H. Kaufman. 1981. Establishment in culture of pluripotential cells from mouse embryos. *Nature* 292 (5819): 154–156.

Folch, A., A. Ayon, O. Hurtado, M. A. Schmidt, and M. Toner. 1999. Molding of deep polydimethylsiloxane microstructures for microfluidics and biological applications. *Journal of Biomechanical Engineering* 121 (1): 28–34.

Folch, A., and M. Toner. 1998. Cellular micropatterns on biocompatible materials. *Biotechnology Progress* 14 (3): 388–392.

Hwang, H., G. Kang, J. H. Yeon, Y. Nam, and J. K. Park. 2009. Direct rapid prototyping of PDMS from a photomask film for micropatterning of biomolecules and cells. *Lab Chip* 9 (1): 167–170.

Martin, G. R. 1981. Isolation of a pluripotent cell line from early mouse embryos cultured in medium conditioned by teratocarcinoma stem cells. *Proceedings of National Academy of Sciences USA* 78 (12): 7634–7638.

Peerani, R. 2008. Engineering the embryonic stem cell niche to control cell fate. *Chemical Engineering and Applied Chemistry,* Toronto, Canada.

Peerani, R., K. Onishi, A. Mahdavi, E. Kumacheva, and P. W. Zandstra. 2009. Manipulation of signaling thresholds in "engineered stem cell niches" identifies design criteria for pluripotent stem cell screens. *PLoS One* 4 (7): e6438.

Williams, R. L., D. J. Hilton, S. Pease, T. A. Willson, C. L. Stewart, D. P. Gearing, E. F. Wagner, D. Metcalf, N. A. Nicola, and N. M. Gough. 1988. Myeloid leukemia inhibitory factor maintains the developmental potential of embryonic stem cells. *Nature* 336 (6200): 684–687.

Zandstra, P. W. 2004. The opportunity of stem cell bioengineering. *Biotechnology and Bioengineering* 88 (3): 263.

Zhong, Z., Z. Wen, and J. E. Darnell, Jr. 1994. Stat3: A STAT family member activated by tyrosine phosphorylation in response to epidermal growth factor and interleukin-6. *Science* 264 (5155): 95–98.

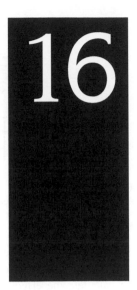

The Fahraeus–Lindqvist Effect
Using Microchannels to Observe Small Vessel Hemodynamics

16.1 Background

Bioengineered tissues and cells are highly dependent upon the surrounding micro-environment for oxygen and nutrient supply as well as waste removal. Organs and thicker tissues require an extensive branching network of blood vessels to perform these same functions, particularly for maintenance of cells at the center of the organ or tissue. Therefore, hemodynamics (study of blood flow) and examination of blood composition are of significant interest to bioengineers who are designing tissue-engineered medical products (TEMPs) or modeling blood flow patterns in vivo.

Blood is a "fluid tissue" of nonhomogeneous composition; blood cells are suspended in protein-enriched plasma that circulates throughout the body via a complex network of vessels. The volume fraction of red blood cells (RBCs) in blood is known as the hematocrit. Because RBCs are directly responsible for oxygen delivery and gas exchange, hematocrit and the blood flow rate directly impact efficiency of gas exchange. The cellular component of blood also includes leukocytes (white blood cells), which play an important role in the immune response. In general, the viscosity of blood is dependent on the cellular concentration and will consequently affect the nature of blood flow, including flow rate, flow profile, etc. Certain pathological conditions, such as sickle cell anemia, in which RBC abnormalities cause cell stiffening and clumping, exhibit higher effective blood viscosity and subsequently altered flow.

The Fahraeus–Lindqvist (F–L) effect describes how the viscosity of blood changes as the diameter of the vessel through which it travels also changes (Fahraeus and Lindqvist 1931). Specifically, studying flow in vessels less than 250 μm in diameter, it was determined that blood has a lower effective viscosity in smaller vessels

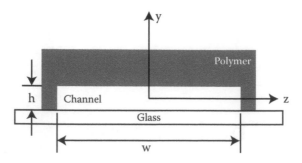

Figure 16.1
Cross section of a typical rectangular microchannel of width w and height h. The channels are constructed from a polymer cast bonded to a glass slide. The coordinate axes y and z are referred to in Equation 16.4.

and hematocrit is reduced as vessel diameter decreases. Fahraeus and Lindqvist used fine glass capillaries with circular cross sections to perform their experiments. To calculate the effective viscosity, μ_{eff}, in their conduits, they used the classical Poiseuille law:

$$Q = \frac{\pi R^4}{8\mu_{eff}} \frac{\Delta P}{L}$$ (16.1)

where
Q is the flow rate
R is the capillary radius
ΔP is the pressure drop across the capillary
L is the capillary length

However, for channels of rectangular cross section such as those used in this and other blood flow laboratory protocols, the equation takes on a slightly different form to account for the change in geometry (Young and Simmons 2009). The accepted form of the equation for rectangular conduits is

$$u_m = \frac{2}{\beta} \frac{D_h^2}{\mu_{eff}} \frac{\Delta P}{L}$$ (16.2)

In this equation, $u_m = Q/A$ is the mean velocity in the rectangular channel of cross-sectional area A (A = width, w, × height, h) (Figure 16.1). The capillary radius R of Equation 16.1 is replaced by the hydraulic diameter defined as $D_h = 4A/P_w$, where P_w is the wetted perimeter—$2(w + h)$—or the total length of the four sides of the rectangle. Finally, β is a constant relating the friction factor f of the channel and the Reynolds number Re and is given by the following empirical relationship for channel aspect ratio $\alpha = h/w$:

$$\beta = f \cdot Re = 96[1 - 1.3553\alpha + 1.9467\alpha^2 - 1.7012\alpha^3 + 0.9564\alpha^4 - 0.2537\alpha^5] \quad (16.3)$$

For gravity-driven flow, the pressure drop across the channel can be predicted by $\Delta P = \rho g H$, where H is the height difference from inlet to outlet reservoir. Therefore, the measurement of mean velocity in the microchannel provides a solution to the effective viscosity using Equation 16.2.

For laminar flow in rectangular channels, a theoretical solution is available that requires Fourier series expansions. For convenience, however, a much simpler formula was proposed by Purday (1949; Shah and London 1978). For a microchannel of half-width ($a = w/2$) and half-height ($b = h/2$), the laminar velocity profile through a rectangular cross section can be approximated by

$$\frac{u}{u_m} = \left(\frac{m+1}{m}\right)\left(\frac{n+1}{n}\right)\left[1 - \left(\frac{y}{b}\right)^n\right]\left[1 - \left(\frac{z}{a}\right)^m\right] \quad (16.4)$$

and

$$\frac{u_{max}}{u_m} = \left(\frac{m+1}{m}\right)\left(\frac{n+1}{n}\right) \quad (16.5)$$

where u and u_{max} are the local axial and maximum velocities, respectively, and m and n are empirical parameters governed by

$$m = 1.7 + 0.5\alpha^{-1.4} \quad (16.6)$$

and

$$n = \begin{cases} 2 & \alpha \leq 1/3 \\ 2 + 0.3(\alpha - 1/3) & \alpha > 1/3 \end{cases} \quad (16.7)$$

The velocity profile of Equation 16.4 is illustrated in Figure 16.2. The profile is parabolic in the y-direction. Maximum velocity occurs at the midplane at $y = 0$ and is fairly constant throughout the midplane except near the side walls.

In normal mammalian blood, the cell density (hematocrit) is ~45%. This value can be easily verified by a simple calculation using known information:

5×10^6 RBCs/mm^3 = 5×10^6 RBCs/μL = 5×10 RBCs/mL blood (Hall 2011)

Volume of one RBC = 98 μm^3 (Ethier and Simmons 2007)

Volume of RBCs per milliliter of blood = 5×10^9 RBCs/mL $\times$ 98 μm^3 = 0.49 mL RBCs/ mL blood

0.49 mL RBCs/mL blood = 49% hematocrit

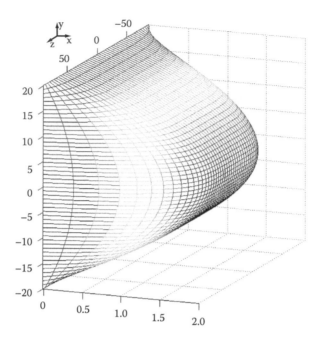

Figure 16.2
Parabolic velocity profile in a rectangular channel (from Equation 16.4).

Similar calculations can be performed to determine the cell density for any cell suspension in microchannels. For this lab, L929 mouse fibroblasts are used to examine fluid flow. Assume that these cells are spherical while in suspension with a diameter $(d) \sim 16.5$ μm.

Velocity in the microchannel must be known in order to determine effective viscosity, μ_{eff}. The most convenient way to measure velocity is by particle streak velocimetry. Briefly, particles traveling at a steady velocity (u) generate a streak line in flow of length l over time t (Figure 16.3). Measuring the length of streak lines in an image taken at a given exposure time yields velocity $u = l/t$. However, particles can reside on different streamlines of flow and streak lines may have different lengths depending on the particle's location. If one takes care to focus on the channel mid-plane during experimentation to take measurements of the longest streak lines, reasonably accurate measurements of the maximum channel velocity can be obtained. Using the velocity profile of Equation 16.4 and the approximate solution to u_{max} in Equation 16.5, one can determine the mean velocity u_m and, ultimately, μ_{eff}.

16.2 Learning Objectives

The objectives of this experiment are to

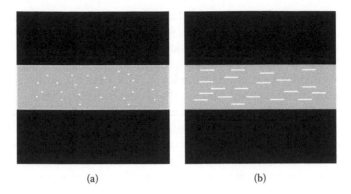

(a) (b)

Figure 16.3
Representations of particle streak velocity images. Streak lines demonstrated in (a) are visible at short exposure time and are suitable for determining cell density. Streak lines represented in (b) are acquired at longer exposure times and are suitable for determining velocity.

- Observe the effect of microchannel (or capillary) dimensions on the viscosity and cell density (i.e., hematocrit) of a given cell suspension flow through the microchannel
- Measure effective viscosity as a function of microchannel width
- Measure microchannel relative cell density (i.e., relative tube hematocrit) as a function of microchannel width
- Discuss sources of error of the current setup compared to the original Fahraeus–Lindqvist setup
- Evaluate the applicability of the current experimental setup as a suitable modified version of the original Fahraeus–Lindqvist setup

16.3 Overview of Experiment

This lab attempts to reproduce the results obtained by Fahraeus and Lindqvist in their experiments on blood flow in small-diameter capillaries. They observed two somewhat surprising phenomena:

- Effective viscosity of blood decreased with decreasing capillary radius.
- The tube hematocrit was always less than the hematocrit in the feed reservoir.

Using the fabrication techniques described in detail in Appendix 5, four microchannels of rectangular cross section were designed and assembled. Briefly, photolithography is used to create a negative relief template, or *master,* consisting of four raised channels with different widths and constant height (Figure 16.4a). Polydimethylsiloxane (PDMS) is cast on this template and polymerized, a technique called soft lithography (Figure 16.4b). Once the PDMS polymerizes, it is peeled away and bonded to a glass slide to form four microchannels (Figure 16.4c). Inlet and outlet ports at the ends of each channel are cored out of the PDMS using a biopsy punch. Syringes, which serve as reservoirs for the cell suspension that will be driven through the microchannels, are attached via tubing (Figure 16.4d).

The microchannels serve as alternative conduits to the capillaries (of circular cross section) used by Fahraeus and Lindqvist. Fibroblasts in suspension will be driven out of the reservoirs and through the microchannels to mimic blood flow through fine capillaries. Images acquired using a CCD camera mounted on a light microscope system will be used to determine microchannel cell density (by cell counting) and analysis of suspension flow rate by particle streak velocimetry. *Note: Chapter 3 of* Introductory Biomechanics *by Ethier and Simmons (2007) provides a thorough review of hemodynamics and blood rheology and is recommended background reading for this experiment.*

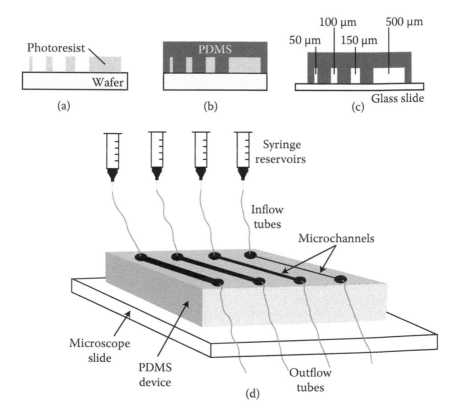

Figure 16.4
Schematic of fabrication of the microchannel device used in this experiment. (a) Photolithography is used to create a master consisting of four raised channels with different widths and constant height. (b) PDMS is cast on this template and polymerized. (c) Once the PDMS polymerizes, it is peeled away and bonded to a glass slide to form four microchannels. (d) Inlet and outlet ports at the ends of each channel are cored out of the PDMS using a biopsy punch. Flow through each microchannel is controlled independently by a syringe reservoir and inlet/outlet tubing.

16.4 Safety Notes

Handle microchannel devices carefully as the glass slides can easily break. Although they have blunt ends, the 21-gauge needles attached to cell flow syringes must be handled carefully to avoid injury.

16.5 Materials

In addition to the general equipment and supplies, the following are needed to complete this experiment:

16.5.1 Reagents and Consumables

- L929 Cells in suspension (1–4 mL @ 20×10^6/mL L929 media)
- Four 1 mL syringes (Becton Dickinson Luer-Lok, disposable)
- Four 21-gauge blunt-ended needles (The instructor should prepare blunt-ended needles before the lab session.)
- Polyethylene tubing (e.g., VWR PE60 and PE190; diameter should be matched to needle and inlet and outlet ports)

16.5.2 Equipment and Supplies

- Devices with four microchannels (constant height but varied widths)
- Phase-contrast microscope equipped with camera and automated image acquisition software

16.6 Recipes

L929 Media. Add 50 mL bovine calf serum (BCS) and 5 mL of 100X penicillin/streptomycin (P/S) to 445 mL of high-glucose DMEM.

16.7 Methods

16.7.1 Session 1: Measure Cell Velocity through Microchannels

1. Obtain one microchannel device, four syringes, and four blunt-ended needles from the instructor.
2. Attach a blunt-ended needle to each syringe and then connect one needle to each inlet port of the microchannel device using polyethylene tubing.

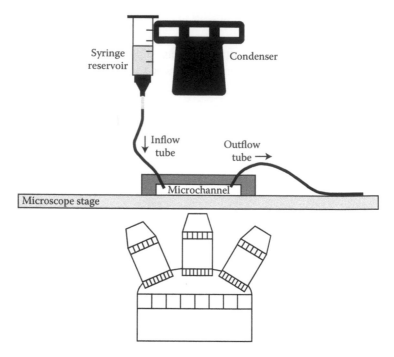

Figure 16.5
Experimental setup. The microchannel device is mounted to the stage of an inverted microscope. The syringe reservoir containing cell suspension is mounted above the stage (i.e., at the level of the condenser) to create gravity-driven fluid flow.

3. Mount the device to the stage of the microscope system (Figure 16.5). At this time, do not mount a syringe onto the condenser as shown in the figure.

4. Select an appropriate objective lens and focus on the channel of interest. Remember that you will be examining cell flow through all four channels for flow rate comparison.

5. Set up the camera software. You will need to acquire images in "live" mode.

6. Make appropriate adjustments to the light intensity and focus to obtain a clear image on the monitor. Depending on the parfocality of the system, the field of view may not be in focus through both the microscope eyepieces and on the monitor at the same time. For experimental purposes, ensure that there is good focus on the monitor.

7. Practice using the software to acquire five images using short exposure time (e.g., 3 ms).

8. Once acquisition settings on the software have been determined, you may begin the experiment.

9. Remove the plunger from one of the syringes. Use a micropipette to load cell suspension into the syringe barrel. Gently reattach the plunger to the syringe and apply slight force to push the cell suspension into the microchannel. When the channel is loaded with cells, quickly remove the plunger. *Note: Using an open syringe as a reservoir to create a gravity head is a reliable and simple method to generate pressure-driven flow; however, the pressure provided by gravity is insufficient to overcome the resistance of the tubes and channels. A slight pressure on the plunger of the syringe will*

overcome this resistance, but continued application of force would alter the pressure and affect velocity.

10. Using lab tape, attach the syringe containing cell suspension to the microscope such that it sits ~10–15 cm above the device (Figure 16.5). Recall that this establishes gravity-driven flow in the microchannel.

11. Acquire 5–10 images using short exposure time (e.g., 3 ms). The cells should appear spherical. Remember to save these images as they will be used to count the number of cells per image to determine cell density within the channel.

12. Acquire 5–10 more images using a longer exposure time (e.g., 10 ms). The cells should appear as streaks (Figure 16.3). Make sure to save these images as well, for they will be used to estimate the velocity and flow rate within the microchannel.

13. Once an appropriate number of images has been acquired for cell flow in the first channel, repeat the same procedure for the three remaining channels.

14. Before leaving the lab, obtain a calibration image from the instructor.

16.8 Data Processing

Briefly report the results of your experiment in paragraph and graphical form. Each of the key results to report in text, figure, and/or table format is described next.

1. Using images obtained during the lab and the equations listed in the background section, calculate the estimated relative "tube hematocrit" (cell density within the microchannel) and the effective viscosity of the cell suspension for each of the four microchannels.

2. For direct comparison with Fahraeus and Lindqvist,

   a. Compare the tube hematocrit calculated previously with the "hematocrit" of the cell suspension in the syringe. Comment on how your data compare with that reported in the literature. Refer to Figure 3-16 from Ethier and Simmons (2007) or Figure 2 from Barbee and Cokelet (1971).

   b. Plot your results as effective viscosity versus tube radius. Compare your results to those in the literature. Refer to Figure 3-15 from Ethier and Simmons (2007) or Figure 2 from Haynes (1960).

3. Create a figure comparing acquired images at each exposure time for the four different microchannels. Include scale bars and appropriate labels.

16.9 Prelab Questions

1. Why is such a high concentration of cells required in this experiment?

2. Calculate the hydraulic diameter for each of the microchannels used in this experiment. For this calculation, assume the channels have a height of 60 μm. Obtain the exact channel height from your instructor when you complete the lab.

3. With reference to Equation 16.4, what would you predict happens to the flow velocity as you approach the side walls of the microchannel?

4. Read the information on microfluidic device design and fabrication in Appendix 5. Briefly explain why this experiment is performed with a channel of rectangular, not circular, cross section.

16.10 Postlab Questions

1. Do your results follow the same trends as those observed by Fahraeus and Lindqvist?

2. Briefly describe a follow-up experiment that could be run to generate a curve similar to that shown in Figure 3-15 from Ethier and Simmons (2007) and Figure 2 from Haynes (1960).

3. What are the major differences between the experimental setup in this lab and the original setup of Fahraeus and Lindqvist?

References

Barbee, J. H., and G. R. Cokelet. 1971. The Fahraeus effect. *Microvascular Research* 3 (1): 6–16.

Ethier, C. R., and C. A. Simmons. 2007. *Introductory biomechanics: From cells to organisms.* New York: Cambridge University Press.

Fahraeus, R., and T. Lindqvist. 1931. The viscosity of the blood in narrow capillary tubes. *American Journal of Physiology* 96:562–568.

Hall, J. E. 2011. *Guyton and Hall textbook of medical physiology,* 12th ed. New York: Elsevier.

Haynes, R. H. 1960. Physical basis of the dependence of blood viscosity on tube radius. *American Journal of Physiology* 198:1193–1200.

Purday, H. F. P. 1949. *An introduction to the mechanics of viscous flow: Film lubrication, the flow of heat by conduction, and heat transfer by convection.* New York: Dover Publications, Inc.

Shah, R. K., and A. L. London. 1978. *Laminar flow forced convection in ducts.* New York: Academic Press.

Young, E. W. K., and C. A. Simmons. 2009. "Student lab"-on-a-chip: Integrating low-cost microfluidics into undergraduate teaching labs to study multiphase flow phenomena in small vessels. *Chemical Engineering Education* 43 (3): 232–240.

Chapter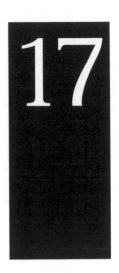

Examining Single-Cell Mechanics Using a Microfluidic Micropipette Aspiration System

17.1 Background

The internal mechanical structure of a cell, the cytoskeleton, consists of a network of actin filaments, intermediate filaments, and microtubules that mechanically support the cell membrane and its contents. These filaments reorganize in response to cell–cell contact, external mechanical forces, and chemical signals, making cells dynamically responsive to their external environment (Chen, Tan, and Tien 2004; Smith et al. 2003; Trickey, Vail, and Guilak 2004). As a consequence of cytoskeletal reorganization, cells may respond by changes in their metabolic activity, cellular adhesion, secretion, or even gene expression (Ingber 2006; Orr et al. 2006). In this manner, the cytoskeleton is considered to function as a mechanotransducer (Wang and Thampatty 2006).

Multiple techniques have been developed to determine the material properties of single cells, including atomic force microscopy (AFM), optical tweezers, compressive testing, and magnetic microbead microrheometry (Ethier and Simmons 2007). All of these techniques require precision and delicate sample handling and are very costly to establish in a laboratory setting. In comparison, micropipette aspiration (MA) is advantageous for mechanical characterization of cells because it is simple and relatively inexpensive and can provide force resolutions as low as piconewtons (Ethier and Simmons 2007).

MA is a common micromanipulation method used to quantify the elastic modulus of cells. The technique uses suction pressure to partially aspirate a free-floating cell sample into a glass micropipette with small internal diameter (1–10 μm— smaller than the diameter of a cell). The micropipette is attached to a manipulator that is capable of moving nonadherent objects in three dimensions with micron-scale precision. Contact between the tip and cell sample is visualized by observation through an associated microscope's field of view.

The ability to create gentle suction pressure changes within the system results from a pressure head that is generated by adjusting the height of an associated liquid reservoir downward. This is represented by

$$\Delta P = \rho g h \tag{17.1}$$

where
ΔP = the pressure difference caused by moving the liquid column
h = the change in height of liquid column
ρ = the density of liquid (1 g/mL for water)
g = the acceleration due to gravity (9.8 m/s²)

For example, lowering the reservoir by 5 cm applies an aspiration pressure of $\Delta P = \rho g h = (1 \text{ g/mL} \times 9.8 \text{ m/s} \times 5 \text{ cm}) = {\sim}0.5$ kPa.

The pressure differential caused by the height of the liquid column aspirates a floating cell into the micropipette (Figure 17.1). The aspiration length (L_A), in conjunction with the applied pressure, can then be used to determine cellular stiffness. While there are a number of analytical models to extract the elastic modulus from these results, the half-space model is the simplest and most common:

$$E = \Phi \times \left(\frac{3r}{2\pi} \right) \times \left(\frac{\Delta P}{L_A} \right) \tag{17.2}$$

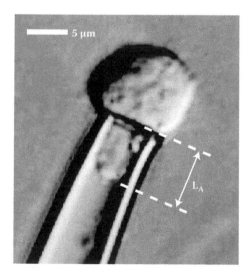

Figure 17.1
Micrograph showing the aspiration length (L_A) of a cell into a micropipette tip.

where

E = Young's modulus

r = pipette radius

L_A = aspiration length

ΔP = change in pressure

Φ = dimensionless constant (Φ depends upon the ratio between pipette wall thickness and pipette radius; a value of 2.1 is taken for most experiments; Theret et al. 1988)

Because it is a specialized piece of equipment, the micromanipulator is the greatest expense associated with this technical setup. A "soft" microdevice, the integrated micropipette aspiration chip (iMAchip), has been developed to make this experimental technique more readily available to research and teaching laboratories (Moraes et al. 2010) (Figure 17.2).

The iMAchip is fabricated using a process called soft lithography, which is described in detail in Appendix 5. Briefly, a Y-shaped channel is fabricated by casting polydimethylsiloxane (PDMS) onto a negative relief template. The PDMS is peeled away and bonded to a glass slide; the resulting channel is ~40 μm in height. A micropipette (inner diameter ~ 5 μm) is carefully placed at the entry of the Y-shaped channel and fixed with epoxy. Standard fluidic port connectors and a three-way valve are used to attach the iMAchip to a pressure-driven syringe and a fluid pressure setup consisting of a height-adjustable reservoir (Figure 17.3). The selector valve can be used to apply two ranges of pressure to the iMAchip. This allows the microchannels to be used for delivery of cells to the micropipette without the use of a micromanipulator.

The advantage of the three-way valve system is the ability to control aspiration pressures. When the valve isolates the *syringe* from the rest of the system, the reservoir can be raised and lowered to apply positive and negative pressures, respectively, to cells being aspirated (Figure 17.4a). This setup is typically used to observe cell deformation once a cell has been "trapped" by the micropipette. The applied

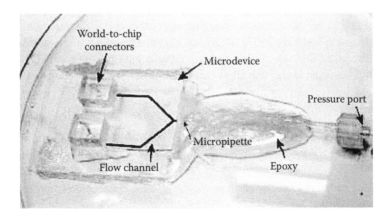

Figure 17.2
Integrated micropipette aspiration chip (iMAchip).

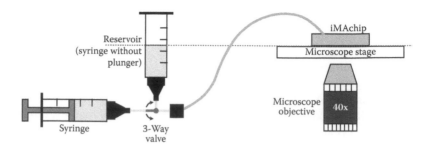

Figure 17.3
Schematic of iMAchip and pressure delivery setup. By changing the height of the reservoir in relation to the microdevice, the applied pressure can be controlled. In the schematic, the liquid level of the reservoir is at the same height as the iMAchip on the microscope stage, the system is in equilibrium, and zero pressure is applied.

pressure depends upon the height of the reservoir in relation to the microdevice: When the liquid level of the reservoir is at the same height as the iMAchip on the microscope stage, the system is in equilibrium and zero pressure is applied.

When the valve isolates the *reservoir* from the rest of the system, the syringe can be used to apply large positive or negative pressures to move cells within the microchannel (Figure 17.4b). This setup is typically used to attract floating cells to the micropipette tip. However, if necessary, this system can also be used to flush cells away from the micropipette. The luer valve stopcock can also isolate the iMAchip from both the reservoir and syringe (Figure 17.4c). This position can be used to fill the syringe from the reservoir. Pumping the syringe in this position will eliminate any bubbles that may have formed. This microdevice platform is capable of performing micropipette aspiration while eliminating the micromanipulator component of the system.

The ability to evaluate single-cell mechanics is an important experimental technique that provides greater insight into how cells receive and integrate regulatory signals from the surrounding environment. This is particularly relevant to understanding disease progression and pathology. However, cytoskeletal changes also alter the mechanical properties of cells at varying stages of stem cell differentiation (Guck et al. 2005; Titushkin and Cho 2007). This may lead to alterations in the normal physiological behavior of these stem cells and can significantly impact normal embryonic development; however, it also can allow direction of tissue regeneration strategies.

17.2 Learning Objectives

The objectives of this experiment are to

- Successfully conduct micropipette aspiration on cells using a microfabricated device
- Determine the Young's modulus of 3T3 fibroblasts
- Quantify the degree of variation within a homogeneous cell population
- Determine sources and the impact of errors associated with this experimental setup

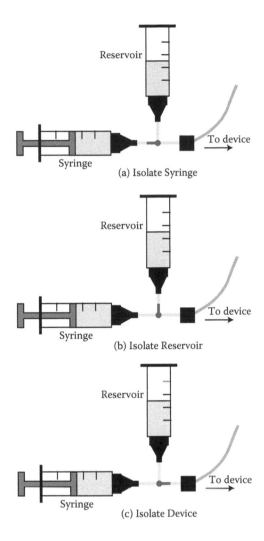

Reservoir

Syringe

To device

(a) Isolate Syringe

Reservoir

Syringe

To device

(b) Isolate Reservoir

Reservoir

Syringe

To device

(c) Isolate Device

Figure 17.4
The three-way valve controls which elements in the experimental setup (syringe, reservoir, or device) are connected. To isolate one element, turn the valve so that the longest part of the knob points toward that element. (a) When the valve isolates the syringe, the device is connected to the reservoir. (b) When the valve isolates the reservoir, the device is connected to the syringe. (c) When the valve isolates the device, the reservoir and syringe are connected.

17.3 Overview of Experiment

The Young's modulus of 3T3 fibroblast cells will be examined using a modified version of a microaspiration system. The iMAchip micropipette aspirator is a microdevice platform mounted on the stage of a microscope with image acquisition capability. The device is connected to a height-adjustable media reservoir that allows pressure-driven delivery of cell-containing media into the device. An associated syringe is used to apply negative and positive pressures to draw single cells to the micropipette tip. Quickly switching the pressure setup to the reservoir will induce mechanical force and promote cell deformation, which can be recorded and consequently measured.

17.4 Safety Notes

Use caution when working with microfluidic devices. The glass slides must be handled carefully because they are susceptible to breaking.

17.5 Materials

In addition to the general equipment and supplies, the following are needed to complete this experiment:

17.5.1 Reagents and Consumables

- 3T3 Fibroblasts in suspension (≥50 μL @ 1×10^6/mL 3T3 media) (Any cell type with a diameter > 10 μm when in suspension will work in this experiment.)
- 3T3 Media
- DMEM (serum free)
- 60 mL Reservoir syringe (plunger removed)
- 10 mL Syringe
- 1/16 in. ID PVC tubing
- Three-way valve
- Assortment of tubing fittings

17.5.2 Equipment and Supplies

- iMAchip microdevice
- Standard ruler
- Retort stand and clamp to position reservoir
- Pipetting bulb

17.6 Recipes

3T3 Media. Add 50 mL bovine calf serum (BCS) and 5 mL of 100X penicillin/streptomycin (P/S) to 445 mL of DMEM (high glucose).

17.7 Methods

17.7.1 Session 1: Perform Micropipette Aspiration

1. Place the iMAchip microdevice on the stage of the microscope acquisition system.

2. Using tubing and connectors, attach the reservoir (60 mL syringe without the plunger) and syringe to the three-way valve as shown in Figure 17.3. Mount the reservoir on a stand using a clamp or rubber bands.

3. Fill the reservoir with DMEM (serum free).

4. Familiarize yourself with the camera settings. Obtain a clear image of the micropipette using the 40X objective lens.

5. Obtain a calibration image from the instructor. Using ImageJ, the diameter of the micropipette can be determined by analyzing the image of the micropipette and the calibration image.

6. Isolate the device from the reservoir and syringe (Figure 17.4c).

7. Fill the syringe halfway with DMEM. Pump if necessary to remove air bubbles.

8. Set the fluid level of the reservoir to 2–3 mm lower than the microscope stage. This will apply an initial tare pressure to the cells to seal a cell to the pipette. Be approximate with the positioning but record the exact height difference. There may be a requirement to play with the initial tare pressure to determine which value works best for this setup.

9. Isolate the reservoir from the syringe and device (Figure 17.4b).

10. Flush the cell suspension into the channels of the device. Do this *slowly* to prevent trapping of air bubbles.

    a. Mix the cell suspension thoroughly by gently pipetting up and down.

    b. Pipette 10 μL of cell suspension into one of the arm ports of the Y-channel (Figure 17.5a).

    c. Place a pipetting bulb securely around the port and gently press down to maintain a seal (Figure 17.5b).

    d. Gently squeeze the bulb to drive fluid through the channels (Figure 17.5c).

    e. Remove the bulb. The channel is now filled with cell-containing media (Figure 17.5d).

11. Add a small volume of cell suspension to the opposite arm port to balance the ports and reach flow equilibrium more quickly.

12. Use the syringe to apply negative and positive pressure in an attempt to draw a cell close to the micropipette tip. *This will take practice!*

13. Avoid dead cells and cells that exhibit membrane blebbing (Figure 17.6).

14. Bring a cell into contact with the micropipette tip.

15. As quickly as possible, switch the valve so that the device is connected to the reservoir rather than the syringe.

16. The cell will equilibrate to the tare pressure in ~30–60 s. Observe deformation of the cell and record an image when the cell does not appear to deform any longer.

17. Apply a negative pressure by lowering the reservoir by ~5 cm.

18. Record the exact height to which the reservoir is lowered.

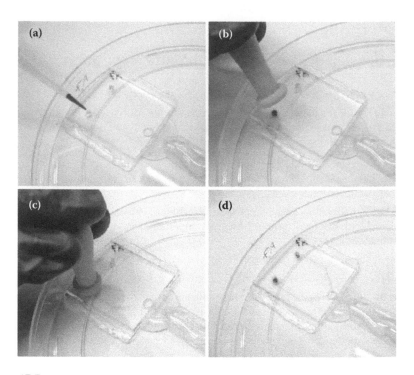

Figure 17.5
Technique for driving the cell suspension through the microchannel. (From Moraes, C. et al. 2010. *Cellular and Molecular Bioengineering* 3 (3): 319–330. With permission.)

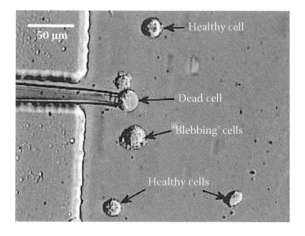

Figure 17.6
Micrograph showing different cellular phenotypes. Avoid making measurements on dead cells or cells that exhibit membrane blebbing.

19. Over the next 90–120 s, the cell will deform into the tip of the micropipette. Because the cell remodels itself in response to these mechanical forces, it may continue to extend very slowly into the pipette (even after 90 s).

20. Record an image once the rate of deformation has become very low (i.e., the cell has reached equilibrium with the new pressure).

21. Switch the pressure setup from the reservoir to the syringe.

22. Blow the cell away from the micropipette tip. Attempt to attract another cell.

23. Reset the reservoir height to a new tare pressure. Repeat the procedure for a different cell.

24. Obtain data for a minimum of five cells.

25. To wash the channel after an experiment, pipette 10 μL of deionized water into one of the ports and push it through using the bulb as described before.

26. Use a lab tissue to wick fluid away from the other port. *Note: Be sure to evacuate the channel of all liquid before flushing in a new cell suspension. This will prevent mixing of cell suspension with water, which will change the osmolarity of the fluid. Force air through the channel and use a lab tissue to wick away any remaining liquid.*

17.7.2 Troubleshooting

If a cell becomes stuck to the micropipette or becomes deflated, suction greater than that provided by the gravity head may be required. The following describes how to set up an alternative and temporary vacuum system for use in these circumstances:

1. If there is no fluid in the syringe, change the valve from the position that isolates the syringe to the position that isolates iMAchip from the reservoir and syringe. Draw fluid from the reservoir into the syringe by pulling the plunger of the syringe.

2. Turn the valve to isolate the reservoir. The iMAchip is now connected to the syringe. To flush the chip, push the plunger. To aspirate, pull the plunger.

3. Once the pipette is cleared, use the syringe to attract a cell as before and then turn the valve to isolate the syringe to control the pressure by the reservoir fluid height.

17.8 Data Processing

Briefly report the results of your experiment as described next.

1. Use the half-space model (Equation 17.2) to analyze the resulting data. A value of 2.1 should be used for Φ in this laboratory. Describe the calculations and show one example in your report.

2. Report the average, standard deviation, and sample size (should be 5 or more).

17.9 Prelab Questions

1. What structures within the cell will determine its mechanical properties, like Young's modulus?

2. What is the advantage of applying the suction pressure by moving the fluid reservoir vertically versus using the syringe?

3. During aspiration of the cell, you will observe the aspiration length to increase even though the applied pressure is held constant. Why does this occur?

17.10 Postlab Questions

1. What are the assumptions of the half-space model?

2. Based on your observations in this lab, are the half-space model assumptions valid?

3. What sources of error are present in the current iMAchip experimental setup? What is the relevant impact of these sources on the results for cellular stiffness?

References

Chen, C. S., J. Tan, and J. Tien. 2004. Mechanotransduction at cell–matrix and cell–cell contacts. *Annual Review of Biomedical Engineering* 6:275–302.

Ethier, C. R., and C. A. Simmons. 2007. *Introductory biomechanics: From cells to organisms.* New York: Cambridge University Press.

Guck, J., S. Schinkinger, B. Lincoln, F. Wottawah, S. Ebert, M. Romeyke, D. Lenz, et al. 2005. Optical deformability as an inherent cell marker for testing malignant transformation and metastatic competence. *Biophysical Journal* 88 (5): 3689–3698.

Ingber, D. E. 2006. Cellular mechanotransduction: Putting all the pieces together again. *FASEB Journal* 20 (7): 811–827.

Moraes, C., K. Wyss, E. Brisson, B. A. Keith, Y. Sun, and C. A. Simmons. 2010. An undergraduate lab (on-a-chip): Probing single cell mechanics on a microfluidic platform. *Cellular and Molecular Bioengineering* 3 (3): 319–330.

Orr, A. W., B. P. Helmke, B. R. Blackman, and M. A. Schwartz. 2006. Mechanisms of mechanotransduction. *Developmental Cell* 10 (1): 11–20.

Smith, P. G., L. Deng, J. J. Fredberg, and G. N. Maksym. 2003. Mechanical strain increases cell stiffness through cytoskeletal filament reorganization. *American Journal of Physiology Lung Cell Molecular Physiology* 285 (2): L456–L463.

Theret, D. P., M. J. Levesque, M. Sato, R. M. Nerem, and L. T. Wheeler. 1988. The application of a homogeneous half-space model in the analysis of endothelial cell micropipette measurements. *Journal of Biomechanical Engineering* 110 (3): 190–199.

Titushkin, I., and M. Cho. 2007. Modulation of cellular mechanics during osteogenic differentiation of human mesenchymal stem cells. *Biophysics Journal* 93 (10): 3693–3702.

Trickey, W. R., T. P. Vail, and F. Guilak. 2004. The role of the cytoskeleton in the viscoelastic properties of human articular chondrocytes. *Journal of Orthopedic Research* 22 (1): 131–139.

Wang, J. H., and B. P. Thampatty. 2006. An introductory review of cell mechanobiology. *Biomechanical Models in Mechanobiology* 5 (1): 1–16.

Chapter **18**

Contribution of Tissue Composition to Bone Material Properties

18.1 Background

Bone is a unique connective tissue consisting of cells embedded within an extracellular matrix composed of an organic, collagen-based component providing ductility (the ability of a solid material to withstand plastic deformation without failure), as well as a mineral hydroxyapatite phase that provides the characteristic rigidity and strength. Bone is continually remodeled throughout one's lifetime, and it has been estimated that approximately 10%–15% of bone throughout the body is replaced with new bone every year (Parfitt 1983). Bone tissue is organized into cortical and trabecular architectures that are distinct based on their degree of porosity (Figure 18.1).

Cortical bone (also known as compact bone) lines the exterior surface of most bones. In cortical bone, the bone tissue is organized into cylindrical structures known as osteons that are composed of concentric lamellae, or plates of bone. Due to its low porosity, cortical bone tends to be stronger and heavier than trabecular bone (also called spongy or cancellous bone). Trabecular bone is found in vertebrae and at the ends of long bones, and is organized into trabecules (struts), which provide trabecular bone with its characteristic porous structure. The higher porosity makes it lighter and somewhat weaker than cortical bone, with a strong correlation between mechanical properties and the degree of porosity (Ethier and Simmons 2007). Consequently, the microarchitecture of bone plays an important role in determining its mechanical properties.

Bone diseases associated with increases in porosity, particularly in trabecular bone, can significantly impact human health and well-being. Weakened bones lead to fracture and often result in reduced mobility, lost productivity, impaired quality of life, and, in some cases, hospitalization. Bone strength is directly affected by bone mineral density and geometry, which are subsequently determined by genetics and disease processes associated with aging. Osteoporosis is characterized by low bone

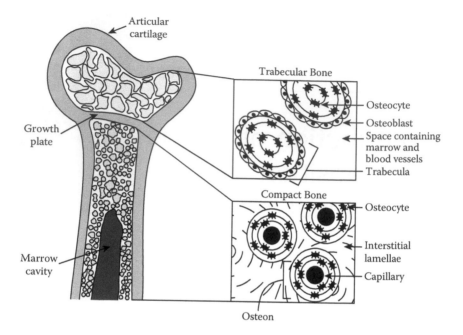

Figure 18.1
Anatomical structure of bone. Insets reveal details regarding the layered nature of the different types of bone. Greater porosity of trabecular bone is evident by the spaced nature of trabeculae. In contrast, reduced porosity of cortical bone is evident by the lamellar structure of osteons within an interstitium.

mass and deterioration of bone at the microscopic level (Ethier and Simmons 2007). The progressive reduction in porosity of trabecular bone leads to smaller and weaker microstructural struts, and therefore osteoporosis sufferers are often unknowingly at increased risk of fragility and bone fracture due to the lack of visible symptoms.

In comparison, bone fragility associated with osteogenesis imperfecta (OI) is due to a genetic defect of collagen type I (Byers and Steiner 1992). Mild forms of OI can result from reduced synthesis of collagen by bone cells, while more serious forms of the disease result from glycine substitutions of certain amino acids. These substitutions damage the ability of collagen molecules to form stable triple helices and, as a consequence, collagen fibrils that contribute to bone strength and ductility are unable to form (Byers, Wallis, and Willing 1991). The loss of these tensile elements in bone contributes to the high incidence of bone fracture among individuals with OI (Falvo, Root, and Bullough 1974).

In order to calculate the material properties of different bone samples within a laboratory setting, a three-point flexural bending test can be performed (Figure 18.2). Bone samples are supported at each end while a constant-rate load is applied at the midpoint (P). As a consequence, uniform deflection occurs on both sides of the loading source.

Maximum stress in the bone under three-point loading occurs at the outer edge directly under the load source. The bending stress at this point is given by

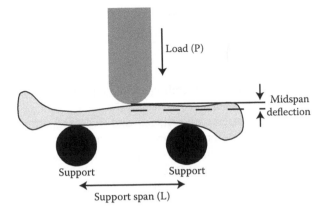

Figure 18.2
A three-point flexural bending test is used to determine the mechanical properties of a bone. The sample is supported equally at each end (support span L) while a constant-rate load is applied at the midpoint (P).

$$\sigma_{bending} = \frac{PLr_o}{\pi(r_o^4 - r_i^4)} \tag{18.1}$$

where
P = load
L = support span
r_o = outer radius of bone at middle
r_i = inner radius of bone at middle

Strain in the bone due to bending (for small deflections only) is given by

$$\varepsilon_{bending} = \frac{12r_o\delta}{L^2} \tag{18.2}$$

where δ is the midspan deflection.

Young's modulus (E) describes the inherent elasticity of a material and is defined as the ratio of stress to strain in the linear elastic region for a material. Young's modulus due to bending is given by

$$E = \frac{PL^3}{12\pi(r_o^4 - r_i^4)\delta} \tag{18.3}$$

The strain energy density of a material is a general measure of the amount of energy absorbed by that material (per unit volume) before failure occurs (i.e., material toughness). The equation for strain energy density (U) is given by

$$U = \int_{0}^{\varepsilon_{failure}} \sigma \, d\varepsilon \tag{18.4}$$

In combination, application of the preceding simple equations can help assess the material properties of a bone sample.

This lab analyzes the effects of collagen and hydroxyapatite on the material properties of bone. These properties are used to model bone diseases such as osteoporosis and OI to develop an understanding of how bone composition and microarchitecture contribute to bone stiffness and strength. These fundamental biomechanical properties must be taken into consideration during the repair and treatment of fractures, as well as during regeneration strategies. Specifically, significant research focuses on the development of scaffolds for use in regeneration of bone tissue for load-bearing situations, as well as for application and development of osteoimplants. As a consequence, engineering of bone tissue also leads to development of new methods for examining and manipulating bone in order to reverse or prevent microarchitectural deficiencies.

18.2 Learning Objectives

The objectives of this experiment are to

- Understand the relationship between calcium and collagen content and the material properties of chicken wing bones under three-point flexural bending
- Discuss the differences and sources of error in using chicken bones to model human bone diseases, such as osteoporosis and OI
- Discuss limitations of this type of testing equipment and protocol

18.3 Overview of Experiment

Chicken wing bones (radii and ulnae) will be prepared in advance by the instructor. The bones will be cut at the ends to remove the marrow and will be measured for mass and volume determination. The class will be divided into several test groups and, prior to measuring mechanical properties, will soak bones in one of the following conditions: water (control, 24 h), vinegar (24 h), or bleach (1 h). Changes in bone density will be determined and recorded pre- and post-treatment. In order to calculate the material properties of the chicken bones, a three-point flexural bending test machine will be used (Figure 18.3). *Note: Prepare the bone samples no more than a day or two before the first experimental session. All bone samples should be stored in vials of water to maintain moisture content and reduce odor.*

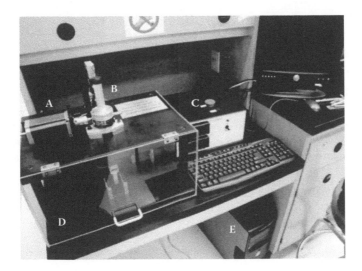

Figure 18.3
Sample bone property testing apparatus. Because material testing instruments can be extremely costly, an alternative is a "home-built" instrument. The apparatus shown here is used at the IBBME Undergraduate Teaching Laboratory (built by Tomas Bernreiter, Department of Mechanical and Industrial Engineering, University of Toronto). A = stepper motor; B = screw jack; C = control box with emergency stop button; D = protective shield; E = data acquisition system.

18.4 Safety Notes

Safety glasses, a lab coat, and gloves should be worn at all times during the lab, particularly when handling bones. Be particularly careful to wear safety glasses when observing mechanical bone testing.

18.5 Materials

In addition to the general equipment and supplies, the following are needed to complete this experiment:

18.5.1 Reagents and Disposables

- Chicken bones (i.e., from wings: radii and ulnae) *Note: Prior to the lab, instructors will prepare bone samples by removing the surrounding meat, thoroughly washing the bones, cutting the ends off, and removing the marrow.*
- Household vinegar
- Household bleach

18.5.2 Equipment and Supplies

- Vernier calipers
- Isomet low-speed bone saw with diamond wafer blade or Dremel tool
- Small metal rod (~3 mm; e.g., small hex key)
- Bone testing apparatus and software *Note: Most mechanical engineering, civil engineering, and materials science departments have material test machines on hand; therefore, this may be the most economical choice for instrument use. However, be certain that borrowed systems can accommodate small force applications to maintain accuracy with small samples such as chicken bones.*

18.6 Recipes

5% Bleach. Mix 5 mL of household bleach with 95 mL water.

18.7 Methods

18.7.1 Session 1: Prepare Bone Samples

1. From your instructor, determine the treatment group that your sample has been assigned to. Acquire a bone sample and the appropriate treatment vial (water, vinegar, or bleach) from the TA.

2. Remove the bone sample from its storage vial and dry thoroughly using paper towels.

3. Measure the mass of the bone using a balance. Record this value in your lab notebook. *Note: Ensure that there is no water on the inside or outside of the bone prior to weighing.*

4. Measure the volume of the bone using a graduated cylinder containing tap water. The initial water level should be sufficient so that when the bone is placed into the cylinder, it is completely submerged without overflowing. Using the smallest graduated cylinder to achieve this will provide the most accurate measurement (usually, 20–50 mL cylinders are appropriate). The change in water level following addition of the bone corresponds to the bone volume. Record this value in your lab notebook. *Note: It is important that the marrow has been sufficiently cleaned out of the center of the bone to prevent trapping of air or fluid during this volume measurement.*

5. Remove the bone from the cylinder and dry thoroughly using paper towels.

6. Measure the diameter at the middle of the bone (this value will be used as the diameter of the bone sample). Record this value in your lab notebook.

7. Measure the average wall thickness of the bone using calipers. Record this value in your lab notebook.

8. Follow the treatment procedure assigned to your group, either water for 24 h, vinegar for 24 h, or bleach for 1 h. Immerse your sample in the designated treatment vial. *Note:*

After treatment, the bones should be transferred to water to prevent them from drying out or becoming malodorous. Testing should be performed as soon as possible (1–2 days) after treatment ends.

18.7.2 Session 2: Test Mechanical Properties

1. Remove the bone sample from the treatment vial and dry thoroughly using paper towels.

2. Measure the post-treatment mass of the bone using a balance. Record this value in your lab notebook.

3. Measure the post-treatment volume of each bone using a graduated cylinder as previously described (session 1; step 4.). Record this value in your lab notebook.

4. Measure the post-treatment diameter at the middle of the bone. Record this value in your lab notebook.

5. Measure the average post-treatment wall thickness of the bone using calipers. Record this value in your lab notebook.

6. Add your data for the mass, volume, and dimensions of your bone sample to the class database that the instructor has created (e.g., Excel spreadsheet on lab computer). Save the file. These data will be shared with all members of the class.

7. Familiarize yourself with the bone property testing apparatus prior to starting your test (Figure 18.3).

8. Move the loading nose to the highest position to allow sufficient room to load the sample into the instrument.

9. Load the bone sample into the fixture of the testing apparatus as described by the manufacturer. Align the middle of the sample with the center of the loading nose (Figure 18.4).

10. The following parameters are recommended for mechanical testing:

    a. Set the test speed (speed at which the loading nose will move downward) to 5 mm/min.

    b. Set sample rate (number of values for load and displacement to be recorded each second) to 10 samples per second.

    c. Ensure that the appropriate parameter is adjusted so that the test ends once the load has dropped to 90% below its peak value.

11. Drop the loading nose so that it is ~1–2 mm above the sample.

12. Be sure to wear safety glasses!

13. Begin the test. The load and displacement curve will be plotted in real time as the test is performed.

14. Ensure that the test is completed before removing the sample. Stop the test prematurely only if large deflections are observed; this will ensure accurate calculations for toughness.

15. Describe the failure (ductile/brittle) and sketch the direction of crack propagation for the bone sample. Record any additional pertinent data regarding the testing.

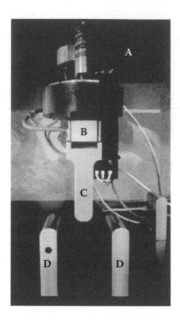

Figure 18.4
Bone property test fixture. Bone samples are placed horizontally on the supports (D) before the loading nose (C) is lowered to exert pressure onto the sample. Load and displacement are measured by transducers (A, B).

16. Save your data. Record all values in your lab notebook or insert a printout of data.

17. Discard bones appropriately once they have been tested.

18. It is recommended to watch testing of other bone samples to observe differences between treatment groups.

19. The instructor will provide data for all treatment groups. Use this collated data for data processing and postlab questions.

18.8 Data Processing

Briefly report the results of your experiment in paragraph and graphical form. Each of the key results to report in text, figure, and/or table format is described next.

1. Create stress–strain graphs due to bending stress (ignore shear effects) for each treatment (water control; vinegar; bleach).

2. Calculate the yield stress, ultimate tensile stress, percentage elongation, and Young's modulus for each treatment. Include a table, similar to Table 18.1, displaying the results of these calculations. Discuss the greatest sources of error in the data.

3. Discuss whether the trends observed for ultimate tensile stress, percentage elongation, and Young's modulus correspond to the expected trends for calcium and collagen deficiency.

TABLE 18.1
Suggested Format for Reporting Data Collected from Mechanical Testing

	Water (24 h)		Vinegar (24 h)		Bleach (1 h)	
	Mean	SD	Mean	SD	Mean	SD
Young's modulus—bending (GPa)						
Peak stress—bending (MPa)						
Peak strain at test end (mm/mm)						
Toughness (MJ/m³)						

4. Plot the Young's modulus versus percentage loss of density for the control (water) and test (vinegar and bleach) bones.

5. Compare the strain energy density of each bone type (use the stress–strain graphs created in part 1) and describe how this property varies with treatment group.

18.9 Prelab Questions

1. Describe the differences between human and chicken bones. Cite your sources.

2. What is the major effect of soaking a bone in vinegar versus soaking a bone in bleach? Cite your sources.

3. Describe other methods of determining long-bone strength. Cite your sources.

18.10 Postlab Questions

1. How could the observed correlation between treatment type and density change be useful clinically?

2. Predict whether this test would be acceptable in modeling osteoporosis and osteogenesis imperfecta in human beings.

References

Byers, P. H., and R. D. Steiner. 1992. Osteogenesis imperfecta. *Annual Review of Medicine* 43:269–282.

Byers, P. H., G. A. Wallis, and M. C. Willing. 1991. Osteogenesis imperfecta: Translation of mutation to phenotype. *Journal of Medical Genetics* 28 (7): 433–442.

Ethier, C. R., and C. A. Simmons. 2007. *Introductory biomechanics: From cells to organisms.* New York: Cambridge University Press.

Falvo, K. A., L. Root, and P. G. Bullough. 1974. Osteogenesis imperfecta: Clinical evaluation and management. *Journal of Bone and Joint Surgery,* American vol. 56 (4): 783–793.

Parfitt, A. M. 1983. The physiologic and clinical significance of bone histomorphometric data. In *Bone histomorphometry,* ed. R. R. Recker. Boca Raton, FL: CRC Press.

Chapter 19

Technical Communication

Presenting Your Findings

19.1 Introduction

It is essential for scientists and engineers to communicate experimental findings to colleagues within their own company and throughout the world. The development of a tissue-engineered medical product is a team effort. To work effectively as a team, there must be good communication among team members and clear documentation of the work that has been completed. To advance technology and scientific knowledge, researchers at one institution must widely disseminate their findings so that those at another institution may build upon the new knowledge.

Two of the methods by which scientists and engineers communicate are probably familiar to you—namely, technical reports and journal articles. These are not the only methods by which results are documented and disseminated. Scientists and engineers often gather at conferences to discuss their work, initiate collaborations, and brainstorm new ideas. It is common for each person presenting at the meeting to contribute an abstract or extended abstract that is distributed to the meeting attendees. It is also common at these meetings for scientists and engineers to display their work in poster format.

This chapter outlines the major components of a technical report or journal article, extended abstract, abstract, and technical poster. The intent is to provide guidelines for reporting your findings to your instructor. Your instructor will specify which format should be used for each experiment. For in-depth coverage of the mechanics of technical writing, see *The Elements of Style* (Strunk 1918), which is available free online, and *Style and Ethics of Communication in Science and Engineering* (Humphrey and Holmes 2008).

19.2 Technical Reports and Journal Articles

The structure and content of technical reports and peer-reviewed journal articles are generally similar and typically contain the following major sections: abstract, introduction, materials and methods, results, discussion, references, and acknowledgments. Carefully review the instructions provided when preparing a report or manuscript for submission to a specific agency or journal because requirements vary. As you read through this section, keep in mind that many of the guidelines for technical reports and journal articles also apply to extended abstracts and posters.

19.2.1 Abstracts

An abstract is a synopsis of work that is typically 250–500 words long, and it is usually the first section in a technical report, journal article, or extended abstract. In this context, it allows the reader to gain an overview of the work quickly and perhaps decide whether or not to read further. An abstract must be very well written to gain the reader's interest. An abstract can also be a stand-alone document, such as when it is published in the proceedings of a conference.

A straightforward approach to writing an abstract is to include one or two sentences for each of the following:

- Background on the topic
- Motivation for the work
- Hypothesis being tested, or objective
- Method or approach used
- Clear statement of the most significant result(s)
- Interpretation of the main result(s)
- Statement of significance of the work

19.2.2 Introduction

The introduction (or background) section of a technical report or journal article provides the reader with the information necessary to comprehend the remainder of the document and establishes the motivation for the work. When considering what information should be included, the author must carefully consider the audience and its familiarity with the topic. For example, an engineer working in a company to develop a blood vessel would not provide information on the structure, function, or composition of vessels when reporting experimental findings to colleagues on the development team. On the other hand, if the same author was preparing a paper for submission to a journal with a wide audience, this information may be necessary to orient the reader to the subject. The level of detail should also be appropriate for the expected readership. With respect to motivating the work within, the introduction should address the importance of the topic, what is currently known in the field, and what information remains unknown (Humphrey and Holmes 2008).

Keep in mind that the introduction is not intended to be a summary of all of the author's knowledge on the subject. Each paragraph should be directly relevant to the content of the report. To ensure that this is the case, it can be helpful to write the introduction after the rest of the report is complete. A typical introduction is three to five paragraphs long and cites relevant literature throughout. *Symbols and abbreviations should be defined the first time they are used and their use should be consistent throughout the document.*

The introduction section usually concludes with a succinct statement of either the objective of the work being reported or the hypothesis of the experiment(s) described within. The objective or hypothesis statement is one of the most, if not *the* most, important sentences in the report. Significant time and multiple revisions are often needed to develop a succinct and precise objective or hypothesis.

19.2.3 Materials and Methods

The purpose of the materials and methods section is to provide the reader with enough information so that he or she could, if needed, replicate the work being reported. It is generally organized into subsections, with each subsection corresponding to a major phase of the work. In this textbook, each lab session could be written up in a separate subsection. The text within materials and methods is dense and an enormous amount of information is conveyed in a minimal amount of space. As you read the scientific literature, pay close attention to how the authors organize and present this information efficiently. Schematics can be very useful for summarizing complex experiments.

Throughout the description of the methods, the author includes the source of any specialized or critical reagents and equipment used. It is common to include the name and location of the manufacturer, in parentheses, immediately following the first mention of the item. Alternatively, this information can be listed in the beginning of the materials and methods section or summarized in the first paragraph. It is sometimes difficult to determine what is considered specialized or critical. Common items such as buffer solutions, ubiquitous chemicals, a standard centrifuge, or incubator would not have a manufacturer listed. On the other hand, the manufacturer is typically reported for reagents where the preparation might affect their function—for example, enzymes, growth factors, or antibodies. This information is also reported for critical equipment.

The materials and methods section typically concludes with a description of the data analysis—in particular, statistical analysis. The author describes the statistical design of the experiment so that the reader can comprehend how conclusions were drawn based on the data. The author should also summarize any calculations performed to analyze the raw data that would not be evident to the reader.

19.2.4 Results

The results section succinctly describes the data collected and objectively presents the results of the subsequent analysis. It is rare to include all the raw data collected in a report. Instead, the analyzed data are condensed in text, table, and/or figure format. In this textbook, however, you are frequently directed to report raw data so that your instructor can verify that the data were analyzed correctly.

19.2.4.1 Reporting Results as Text

Descriptive statistics (e.g., mean, median, percentiles, standard deviation [SD], and standard error of the mean [SEM]) are useful for summarizing data in text format. Recall that mean and SD are appropriate measures of central tendency and variability, respectively, for data drawn from a normally distributed population. For data that are not drawn from a normally distributed population, the median (50th percentile) and other percentiles should be used to describe central tendency and variability. *Note: SEM can be reported instead of SD for normal data if the author wishes to represent the certainty with which the sample estimates the population mean. This is justifiable if the scatter in the data is not particularly meaningful—for example, when it is a measure of experimental error more than biological variability. SEM is not a measure of variability, but SD can be converted to SEM and vice versa as long as the sample size (n) is given.*

Considering the number of options available for reporting data, it is essential to indicate which statistics are reported and provide the corresponding sample size. For example, if you made five independent measurements of a cell suspension on a hemacytometer, you might report that the cell density was $3.2 \times 10^6 \pm 0.5 \times 10^6$ cells/mL (mean $\pm$ SD, $n = 5$). The number of significant digits used should reflect the precision of the measurement while taking into consideration scientific importance. Specifically, you may choose to report fewer significant digits if the precision of the instrument exceeds what is deemed scientifically meaningful. The appropriate units must always be clearly indicated.

Results from statistical analysis are also usually reported in the results section as text. For example, the author may report results of a regression analysis (e.g., coefficient of determination, slope, etc.) or whether samples are significantly different from each other as determined by the appropriate statistical test (t-test, ANOVA, chi-square, etc.) or post hoc test (Bonferroni t-test, Dunnet, Tukey, etc.). If results are statistically different, it is customary to indicate that the associated p-value is <0.05, 0.01, or 0.001, although there is a trend toward reporting precise p-values.

If the results are not statistically different, the statistical power of the test should be reported. This is important because a p-value that exceeds the critical value has two different interpretations. One is that the samples being compared are drawn from the same population (i.e., the treatment tested did not have an effect). The second interpretation is that the samples are from different populations but there were not enough data or the data had too much variability to be able to detect the difference that exists. When reporting results as text, avoid interpretation; succinctly state the result and leave interpretation for the discussion section.

19.2.4.2 Reporting Results in Tables

Tables are useful for organizing a large amount of data that may confuse the reader if presented as text. Tables should be referred to within the text, placed logically within the text, numbered sequentially as they appear, and have a short title. Data within the table should be logically arranged in columns or rows. Formatting is important to identify headings and to help the reader synthesize the information being presented. As is always the case, the number of significant digits should reflect the precision of the measurement while taking into consideration scientific importance. Units are typically indicated following row or column labels (e.g., cell density [cells/milliliter]) so that it is not necessary to repeat the units for each entry in the table.

19.2.4.3 Reporting Results in Figures

Figures, such as images and graphs, are often included to illustrate the most important findings of the study. All figures should be referred to within the text, placed logically within the text, numbered sequentially as they appear, and have a caption.

Images are frequently used to document and communicate qualitative data, such as the micrographs captured in experiments throughout this text. Every micrograph should include an accurate scale bar superimposed on the image. Labels and arrows may also be superimposed on an image to highlight crucial features. Images must be representative of the data they are intended to document and must not be manipulated through image processing methods that compromise interpretation. This is important when acquiring and when analyzing images. For example, if you are collecting images to compare relative intensity of a fluorescent marker (as in Chapter 15), all images must be captured using the same exposure time because increasing exposure time will increase brightness of the image. Similarly, the brightness and contrast of the images should not be altered in postprocessing.

Graphs are often the most effective method of displaying the relationship that exists between quantitative data. There are many different types of graphs and the best choice is often directly related to the design of the experiment. Scatter plots display the relationship between one variable on the x-axis and another on the y-axis. As such, scatter plots are used to display regression or correlation data. When a regression is plotted, the independent variable must be on the x-axis and the dependent variable on the y-axis. When a correlation is plotted, the choice of axis is arbitrary. Bar graphs are useful for displaying similarities or differences that exist among means.

Graphs must include labels and units on each axis, a key that maps experimental groups to the data displayed, and error bars on the data. The caption on a graph should indicate whether the error bars represent SD or SEM and what the sample size is. Typically, results from statistical analysis are displayed directly on the graphs using asterisks to indicate pairwise differences.

Figures are included in reports to communicate important findings—often, the most important findings. Incomplete figures or poor formatting makes it difficult for the reader to understand these. Therefore, time must be invested to make professional quality figures to convey the information effectively and efficiently.

19.2.5 Discussion

The discussion section is the author's opportunity to describe what the results mean and to explain to the reader why the results are important. A simple approach to writing a discussion section is to devote one paragraph (or more, if needed) to each of the following:

- Summary and interpretation of the most important results
- Comparison of your results with those previously reported, including citations to published work
- Discussion of the limitations of the methods used, including sources of error
- Suggestion for future experiments to address these limitations or to extend the findings reported
- Clear statement of the significance of the findings in the context of current knowledge

19.2.6 References

The references section lists all of the publications that are referred to within the technical report or journal article. Cite high-quality references (e.g., books, peer-reviewed publications, etc.) that you have read firsthand and, whenever possible, avoid material published only online. The list of references may be arranged in order of appearance within the text or in alphabetical order. Many formats are acceptable for reporting the source of information; however, it is essential that the references section be complete so that the reader is able to access the cited source. Also, if you are preparing a report or manuscript for submission to a specific agency or journal, carefully review the specific requirements of the agency or journal. Typically, a reference includes author(s), year of publication, title, volume, and page numbers. Use of reference management software can greatly decrease the amount of time needed to prepare the references section and, by allowing the author to download citations directly from the publication, helps avoid citation errors.

19.2.7 Acknowledgments

The authors may use the acknowledgment section to recognize contributions to the work by colleagues who are not included as authors. In the context of this course, you may wish to recognize a teaching assistant who provided extra assistance in completing the experiment or analyzing data. Funding sources, if any, are also typically recognized in the acknowledgments section.

19.3 Extended Abstracts

Scientific conferences often require potential presenters to submit extended abstracts so that the quality and relevance of their work can be assessed in advance of the conference. For example, extended abstracts are required for two meetings that offer special opportunities for undergraduate students: the Annual Meeting of the Biomedical Engineering Society (BMES) and the American Society of Mechanical Engineers (ASME) Summer Bioengineering Conference. An extended abstract is essentially an abbreviated technical report (one to two pages long) divided into the same sections: Abstract, Introduction, Materials and Methods, Results, Discussion, References, and Acknowledgments. The primary content of each section remains unchanged but modifications are made to condense overall length. Do not be deceived by the brevity of an extended abstract; presenting work in this format is often more work than writing a long report since it is time consuming to construct the requisite dense text.

In an extended abstract, the introduction may be reduced from several paragraphs to just one paragraph followed by an objective or hypothesis statement. To accomplish this, emphasis should be placed on providing motivation for the work rather than background information necessary to understand the work. At a scientific conference in your own field, most readers are familiar with the topic. To condense the methods section, it is generally acceptable to make extensive use of familiar abbreviations (e.g., mm for millimeters, min for minute(s), etc.) and even include numbered or bulleted lists. While it may be necessary to leave out some information that would be included in a technical report, the better approach is to condense the information rather than remove it. The description of data analysis is essential and should not be removed.

The results section in a technical report often contains minimal text, so content may not change significantly in an extended abstract. If necessary to save space, results from less significant experiments (e.g., preliminary experiments to determine experimental parameters, validation studies, etc.) may be presented as text rather than as figures, or omitted. *Do not* simply resize figures to fit the condensed format. It is important to maintain the same minimum font size required in the main document within figures so that the information is legible. The discussion section should contain the same elements as in a full technical report; however, each point may be addressed in a few sentences instead of one or two paragraphs. Relevant literature is cited throughout an extended abstract and a list of references, in a very condensed format, is included at the end along with acknowledgments.

If the extended abstract is accepted, the author will present the work at the conference and the extended abstract will be distributed to meeting attendees. As such, most conference planning committees provide a very detailed template so that all the published abstracts conform to the same format. The templates and instructions to authors should be followed *exactly* because submissions are often not edited or revised after the initial submission. Also, reviewers may reasonably conclude that a lack of attention to detail when reporting results may reflect a similar mind-set during execution of the experiments. Your instructor may direct you to use one of these templates to prepare an extended abstract to report your findings in this course.

19.4 Technical Posters

Technical poster sessions are included at many scientific meetings to provide authors an opportunity to speak directly with those interested in their work and to allow a large number of authors to present. The content of a technical poster as illustrated in Figure 19.1 is most similar to that of an extended abstract, although some authors prefer not to include an abstract on posters. Also, the references and acknowledgments sections may be combined to save space. Posters are typically ~36 in. tall × 48 in. wide and are printed on a large-format printer. Specialized publishing software can be used to prepare a poster; however, presentation software (e.g., PowerPoint, Keynote, etc.) also works well. To create a poster using presentation software, open a new document and set the document size to 36 × 48 in. Text and figures can be arranged on the canvas exactly as when making slides. It is a good idea to leave at least 1 in. around the perimeter as a margin. Charges for large-format printing can

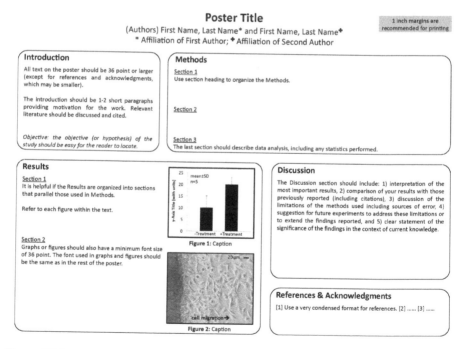

Figure 19.1
Sample layout of a technical poster.

be expensive and are tied to the amount of ink and quality of paper used. To reduce ink use, create your poster on a white background.

Consider the environment in which your poster will be viewed when preparing a technical poster. At conferences, posters are available for viewing throughout the meeting, whether the author is present or not. As such, the poster should be all-inclusive and require no explanation. During designated poster-viewing sessions, authors are present at their poster, but these sessions are frequently very crowded and it is not uncommon to have several people congregated at one poster. In this situation, it is important that all text on the poster be visible from several feet away and that the main point of the work is clear. If not, your colleagues will spend their limited time elsewhere.

References

Humphrey, J. D., and J. W. Holmes. 2008. *Style and ethics of communication in science and engineering.* Princeton, NJ: Morgan & Claypool.

Strunk, W. J., Jr. 1918; 1999 (online). *The elements of style.* Geneva, NY: Press of W. P. Humphrey; Bartleby.com.

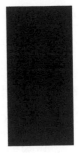

Appendix 1: Trypsinizing a Cell Monolayer

A1.1 Background

Trypsin is a naturally occurring enzyme that cleaves side chains of the amino acids lysine and arginine to break down food in the digestive system. In the lab, the proteolytic activity of trypsin is widely used to disassociate cells growing in monolayer culture. The following protocol can be used whenever it is necessary to release cells from monolayer culture—for example, to subculture or "passage" the cells or to use the cells in an experiment.

A1.2 Safety Notes

Review all relevant MSDSs.

A1.3 Materials

In addition to the general equipment and supplies, the following are needed to complete this protocol:

A1.3.1 Disposables and Consumables

- Cell monolayer
- 0.25% Trypsin with EDTA (1X)
- Complete media (formulation of media depends on the cell type being trypsinized)
- Trypan blue

A1.4 Recipe

Trypsin. Thaw trypsin as supplied, make 2 mL aliquots, store for up to 18 months at –20°C.

A1.5 Methods

1. In a 37°C water bath, warm trypsin and media. Table A1.1 summarizes the volume of trypsin recommended to release cells from common culture vessels. Thaw at least twice the volume needed to release the cells so that the excess can be used for rinsing.

2. Prepare the biosafety cabinet (BSC) for use by wiping it down with 70% ethanol and arranging necessary reagents and disposables.

3. Remove the culture vessel(s) from the incubator, spray lightly with 70% ethanol, and place in the BSC.

4. Aspirate the spent medium from the culture vessel with a Pasteur pipette. Position the Pasteur pipette so the medium is removed without disturbing the cell monolayer.

5. *Quickly* rinse the cell monolayer with half of the trypsin to dilute medium and waste components.

6. *Quickly* and carefully aspirate this rinse solution with a Pasteur pipette.

7. Add the remaining warmed trypsin to the flask. Place the flask in the incubator.

8. Check on the cells after 2–3 min to see if they have detached. *Gently* tap on the side of the flask to release the cells. View cells under the microscope to confirm detachment. Incubate the cells for a few minutes longer if they have not detached. *Avoid exposing cells to trypsin longer than required to release them from the substrate because trypsin will damage cell surface receptors and may slow cell adhesion and spreading.*

9. Add 10 mL of complete media (with serum) to neutralize the trypsin action.

10. Thoroughly rinse the bottom and corners of the flask to release adherent cells.

TABLE A1.1
Recommended Volume of Trypsin to Release a Cell Monolayer from Common Size Flasks and Dishes

Culture Vessel	Approximate Culture Area (cm²)	Recommended Trypsin Volume to Release Cells (mL)	Recommended Trypsin Volume to Thaw (mL)
T25	25	1.0	2.0
T75	75	3.0	6.0
35 mm Dish	10	0.5	1.0
60 mm Dish	21	1.0	2.0
100 mm Dish	57	2.0	4.0

Note: Thaw at least twice the volume needed for the trypsinization so that the excess can be used for the rinse before.

11. Split, concentrate, or use cells as desired:

a. Split the cells by dividing up the cell suspension among multiple culture vessels and then adding media to bring the volume in each vessel up to the working volume. A sample of the cell suspension can be counted using a hemacytometer (see Appendix 2) to determine how to split the cells or a standard "split ratio" can be used. A typical split ratio is 1:10, which means plating the same number of cells on a surface area 10-fold larger then previously. For example, cells from one T75 flask can be replated into ten T75 flasks.

b. To concentrate the cells, spin the suspension down for 5 min in a centrifuge at 250–500 g, discard the supernatant, resuspend the pellet in a small volume of media, count a sample on the hemacytometer, and adjust to desired density.

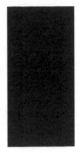

Appendix 2: Counting Cells with a Hemacytometer

A2.1 Background

A hemacytometer is a device used to determine the density of cells within a suspension. It is a thick, glass slide etched with counting grids. A coverslip is placed over the counting grids and a small volume of a cell suspension is injected into the narrow space between. With the aid of a microscope, the number of cells that reside over a defined area of the grid are counted. This cell count can be translated into density within the suspension (in cells/mL) because the dimensions of the counting chamber are known.

While counting cells on a hemacytometer, it is possible to estimate the percentage of viable cells in the whole population by using a stain called trypan blue. This blue dye is actively excluded by living, healthy cells. As such, the cytoplasm of living cells will appear colorless under the microscope. Unhealthy or dead cells are unable to exclude the dye and their cytoplasm will appear dark blue.

A2.2 Safety Notes

Trypan blue is carcinogenic and can be absorbed through skin. Always wear gloves when working with trypan blue. Review all relevant MSDSs.

A2.3 Materials

In addition to the general equipment and supplies, the following are needed to complete this protocol:

A2.3.1 Reagents and Consumables

- Cell suspension (~1×10^6 to 5×10^6 cells/mL)
- Trypan blue

A2.3.2 Equipment and Supplies

- Hemacytometer with coverslip
- Hand tally counter

A2.4 Methods

1. Clean the hemacytometer and cover glass with 70% ethanol. Wipe with a lint-free wiper or blow dry with compressed air. Moisturize the coverslip supports with water and gently place the coverslip on top (this small amount of water will act as an adhesive to hold the coverslip down) before adding cell suspension.

2. Mix the cell suspension with trypan blue:
   a. In the biosafety cabinet, mix the cell suspension thoroughly to break up cell clumps and to obtain a homogenous suspension. Withdraw the entire cell suspension into a serological pipette. Eject the suspension slowly, collecting two samples (one drop each) midstream in separate microfuge tubes. *Note: Sterile microfuge tubes are recommended to avoid contamination of the pipette and, subsequently, the cell suspension.*
   b. Take the microfuge tubes to the lab bench; it is not necessary to keep the samples sterile since they will be discarded after the cells are counted.
   c. In another microfuge tube, mix 40 μL from one of the samples with 10 μL of trypan blue. Repeat with the second sample.

3. Load the cell/trypan blue mixtures into opposite sides on the hemacytometer:
   a. Mix the cells with trypan blue thoroughly by pipetting up and down repeatedly.
   b. Withdraw 10 μL of the first sample into a pipette.
   c. Rest the pipette tip on one of the notches of the hemacytometer.
   d. Gently depress the pipette's plunger, allowing the mixture to flow into the chamber by capillary action. Inject enough to cover the counting surface, but do not allow the chamber to overflow.
   e. Load the counting chamber on the other side with the second cell/trypan blue sample.

4. Count the cells:
   a. Place the hemacytometer on the microscope stage.
   b. Using transmitted light and a low-powered objective (e.g., 10X), adjust the focus and hemacytometer position so that a grid pattern is clearly visible.
   c. With a hand tally counter, count and record the number of *live* cells in the center 25 squares (5 × 5 large squares). This region has an area of 1 mm². To avoid

counting the same cell twice, follow a systematic pattern with your eyes and count cells present on the top and left border but not those on the bottom or right border (Figure A2.1).

d. Count and record the number of *dead* cells in the same region.

e. A good *live* cell count is between 100 and 500 cells. If the cell count is too low, then the sample may not be representative of the cell suspension; if the cell count is too high, it may be difficult to distinguish between neighboring cells. If your

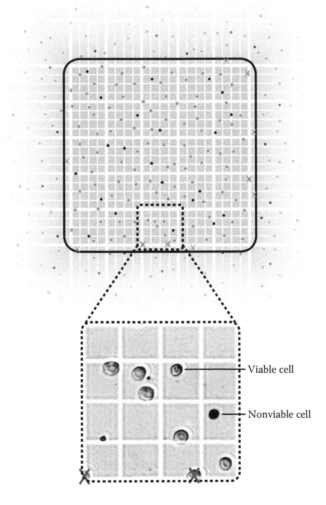

Figure A2.1
Count cells within individual squares and those that touch the left and top borders. Do not count cells that touch the right and bottom borders. The counting should start from the upper right corner and "snake" back and forth until the lower right corner is reached. To determine the percentage of viable cells, count the number of viable and nonviable cells. The percentage of viable cells (82%) is the number of viable cells (98) divided by the total number of cells (120) in the field. The micrograph at the bottom illustrates how viable and nonviable cells appear under the microscope.

count falls well outside this target range, dilute or concentrate the cell suspension as needed and repeat the preceding steps. If your cell count falls within this range, count the second sample, which is already loaded onto the opposite side of the hemacytometer.

5. If the values obtained from the two grids vary significantly (>10%), the original cell suspension may not be evenly mixed and should be recounted. The process should also be repeated if an abundance of clumped cells is visible in the grid. Repeat steps 1–4 until reliable and repeatable counts are obtained. Average the counts.

6. Calculate the percent viability in the cell suspension:

$$\%\text{Viability} = \frac{\text{Live Cell Count}}{(\text{Live Cell Count} + \text{Dead Cell Count})} \times 100\% \qquad (A2.1)$$

7. Calculate the density of cells in the suspension from which the samples were collected (cells per milliliter). Taking the dilution by the trypan blue into consideration, the cell density is

$$\text{Live Cell Density} = 10{,}000 \times 1.25 \times N \qquad (A2.2)$$

where N is the average live cell count from the two samples. *Note: If the live cell density is less than desired, centrifuge the suspension, resuspend the cell pellet in a smaller volume, and repeat the cell counts.*

8. Calculate the total number of live cells in your cell suspension:

$$\text{Total Live Cells} = \text{Live Cell Density} \times \text{Volume of Cell Suspension} \qquad (A2.3)$$

9. Calculate the final suspension volume that will achieve the desired density in the cell suspension (as needed):

$$\text{Final Suspension Volume} = \frac{\text{Total Live Cells}}{\text{Desired Cell Density}} \qquad (A2.4)$$

10. Bring the cell suspension up to the final volume by adding media. Mix well and use the cells as desired.

11. Carefully remove the coverslip and hold it over a trypan blue liquid waste container to spray-wash with 70% ethanol. Spray-wash the chamber slide as well. Use a lab tissue to rub mild detergent gently on the slide and coverslip to remove cellular residue, and then rinse with water followed by deionized water. Place the hemacytometer and coverslip on a lab tissue to dry. Rinse the 0.5 mL microcentrifuge tube with 70% ethanol to remove residual trypan blue (the rinse goes into the trypan blue waste) and discard both this tube and the 1.5 mL microcentrifuge tube containing cell suspension into the biohazard waste.

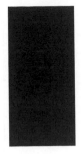

Appendix 3: PicoGreen® DNA Assay

A3.1 Background

Determining the density of cells in a suspension is relatively straightforward using a hemacytometer; however, alternate methods must be used when measuring cell density within a piece of tissue or engineered construct. In these cases, the tissue or scaffold and indwelling cells can be enzymatically digested, mixed with a fluorescent DNA-binding dye, and the fluorescence intensity measured using a fluorometer. A calibration curve is generated from a range of DNA standards to relate the fluorescence intensity of the sample to DNA content. PicoGreen is one of several commercial fluorescent DNA dyes available. The excitation (EX) and emission (EM) spectra for PicoGreen are shown in Figure A3.1.

A3.2 Safety Notes

According to the manufacturer, the mutagenicity and toxicity of PicoGreen have not been assessed. Because this reagent binds to nucleic acids, it should be treated as a potential mutagen, handled with care, and disposed of in accordance with local regulations. Use good lab practices and review all relevant MSDSs.

A3.3 Materials

In addition to the general equipment and supplies, the following are needed to complete this protocol:

A3.3.1 Reagents and Consumables

- Cell or tissue digest
- PicoGreen dsDNA assay kit (including TE buffer and 100 µg/mL DNA standard; Molecular Probes)

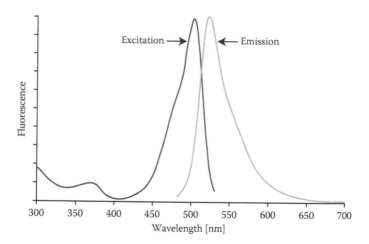

Figure A3.1
Emission (EM) and excitation (EX) spectra for the PicoGreen® DNA-binding dye. Peak excitation and emission are 480 nm and 520 nm, respectively.

A3.3.2 Equipment and Supplies

- Promega Quanti-Fluor fluorometer (EX: 480 nm, EM: 520 nm) with minicell cuvettes
- Vortex mixer

A3.4 Recipes

PicoGreen. Prepare 5 μL aliquots of the 200X stock solution supplied with the PicoGreen kit. Store at –20°C.

TE Buffer. Dilute 20X TE buffer supplied with the PicoGreen kit in deionized water.

100 μg/mL DNA standard. Prepare 5 μL aliquots of the DNA standard supplied with the PicoGreen kit and store at –20°C.

A3.5 Methods

1. Label the microfuge tubes in which you will dilute each standard and sample in preparation for the assay. *Note: Duplicates of the five standards and each sample should be prepared.*

2. Prepare the PicoGreen dye solution:

   a. Determine the total volume of 1X PicoGreen needed. As noted before, each standard or sample should be measured in *duplicate* and each duplicate will be mixed with 50 μL of the dye.

   b. Thaw one 5 μL PicoGreen aliquot per milliliter of dye needed.

   c. Dilute *each* PicoGreen aliquot with 995 μL TE buffer (200-fold dilution).

3. Prepare DNA standards (200–0 ng DNA/mL final volume):

    a. Dilute two 5 μL aliquots of 100 μg/mL DNA to 1 μg/mL with TE buffer (100-fold dilution).

    b. Cap the tubes and vortex the DNA solutions.

    c. Dilute the 1 μg/mL DNA standard solutions into labeled microfuge tubes as shown in Table A3.1. Make two independent sets of standards, one from each solution.

    d. Cap the tubes and vortex each standard.

4. Generate a standard curve:

    a. Turn on and configure the fluorometer to excite at ~480 nm and measure emission at ~520 nm.

    b. Add 50 μL of each standard to a separate minicuvette. Add 50 μL of the PicoGreen dye to each minicuvette. Wait at least 2 min before measuring the fluorescence.

    Note: Carefully vortexing the sample after adding the dye may improve the consistency of the results; however, this should only be done if the sample will not splash out of the cuvette. Tap the cuvette gently on the lab bench to disrupt any air bubbles within the cuvette.

    c. Calibrate the fluorometer according to the manufacturer's instructions.

    d. Measure the fluorescence of each of the standards and verify that the standard curve is approximately linear. If not, try to identify the source of error and repeat until a reliable standard curve is obtained.

5. Prepare samples:

    a. Vortex the samples to mix them well.

    b. Estimate the concentration of DNA in the digest solutions/samples.

    c. In microfuge tubes, dilute a portion of each sample in TE buffer to an approximate concentration of 25–200 ng/mL and a final volume of 250 μL. Repeat so that each dilute sample is prepared in duplicate.

6. Measure DNA content of samples:

    a. Add 50 μL of each sample to separate minicuvettes. Add 50 μL of the PicoGreen dye to each minicuvette. Wait at least 2 min before measuring the fluorescence.

    b. Measure the fluorescence of each sample. If any sample is out of range of the standards or the fluorometer detection limit, dilute the sample more and repeat the

TABLE A3.1
Recipes for Dilution of 1 μg/mL DNA Standard Solution to Generate a Standard Curve

Standard concentration (ng/mL)	200	100	50	25	0
DNA standard solution (1 μg/mL) (μL)	200	100	50	25	0
TE (μL)		300	400	450	475	500

Note: The standards are made up at 2X (twice the desired final concentration) because they will be mixed 1:1 with the PicoGreen dye prior to measurement.

measurement until the reading falls within the working range of the calibration curve. Make careful notes in your lab notebook regarding the dilutions.

A3.6 Data Processing and Reporting

The general approach for analyzing data from the PicoGreen assay is described next. Experiment-specific instructions may also be found in the chapters throughout this text.

1. Enter the fluorescence data and DNA concentrations for the standard curve into Excel or a similar program. Plot these data.

2. Fit a line through the standard data and display the slope, intercept, and r^2 value on the plot. The equation describes the linear relationship between the fluorescence intensity and DNA concentration and the r^2 value describes how strong the relationship is between fluorescence and DNA concentration.

3. Using the preceding equation, determine how much DNA was in each sample within the cuvette.

4. Now account for dilution of the samples (with proteinase-K, TE buffer, and PicoGreen) to determine the original DNA concentration of the samples.

5. If desired, calculate the number of cells per milliliter in the samples based on the amount of DNA per cell. *Note: The quantity of DNA per cell depends on the species from which the sample came.*

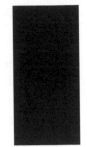

Appendix 4: Dimethylmethylene Blue (DMMB) Assay for Sulfated Glycosaminoglycans

A4.1 Background

Glycosaminoglycans (GAGs) are long, unbranched polysaccharides synthesized by almost all mammalian cells (Varki et al. 2009). GAGs are frequently bound to a core protein, forming a proteoglycan, and are located primarily on the surface of cells or within the extracellular matrix (ECM) (Varki et al. 2009). Specific GAG chains include hyaluronan, chondroitin sulfate, dermatan sulfate, heparan sulfate/heparin, and karatan sulfate. All GAGs, except hyaluronan, contain sulfate groups. Dimethylmethylene blue (DMMB) binds to sulfated GAGs, causing a shift in its absorbance. For nearly 30 years, DMMB has been widely used to measure the concentration of sulfated GAGs in a solution (Farndale, Buttle, and Barrett 1986; Farndale, Sayers, and Barrett 1982). The change of absorbance that accompanies binding of DMMB to GAGs is measured using a spectrophotometer and compared to a calibration curve generated from standards of known GAG concentration.

A4.2 Safety Notes

Use good lab practices and review all relevant MSDSs.

A4.3 Materials

In addition to the general equipment and supplies, the following are needed to complete this experiment:

A4.3.1 Reagents and Consumables

- Sample containing GAGs in solution (e.g., tissue digest)
- Phosphate-buffered EDTA (PBE)
- 10 mg/mL Chondroitin sulfate sodium salt from shark cartilage in PBE (GAG standard)
- Dimethylmethylene blue (DMMB) dye
- Filter paper
- Untreated, flat-bottom, 96-well plate

A4.3.2 Equipment and Supplies

- Amber storage bottle
- Microplate reader (with 525 nm acquisition capability) and acquisition software

A4.4 Recipes

0.1 M Phosphate buffer. Reconstitute according to manufacturer's instructions or purchase 1X solution.

PBE. Dissolve ethylenediaminetetraacetic acid disodium salt dihydrate (EDTA; MW = 372) at 1.86 mg/mL in 0.1 M phosphate buffer, adjust pH to 7.1 with HCl and NaOH, and store at room temperature (RT).

10 mg/mL GAG standard. Dissolve chondroitin sulfate from shark cartilage in PBE at 10 mg/mL, prepare 50 μL aliquots, and store at –20°C.

40 mM Sodium chloride (NaCl) + 40 mM glycine. Dissolve 2.34 g NaCl and 3 g glycine in enough deionized water (dH$_2$O) to bring the total volume to 1 L.

DMMB dye. Dissolve 8.0 mg DMMB in 1 mL ethanol, wrap tube in aluminum foil, and dissolve overnight with stirring. Bring DMMB to 500 mL in NaCl/glycine solution, pH 3.0, and filter into an amber bottle. Check the absorbance of the DMMB solution at 525 nm (A_{525}) using the NaCl/glycine solution as a blank. If the absorbance is >0.32, add more NaCl/glycine solution. Store up to 3 months at RT.

A4.5 Methods

1. Preparation of GAG standards (125–0 μg/mL):
   a. Dilute two 50 μL aliquots of the 10 mg/mL GAG stock to 1 mg/mL with PBE (10-fold dilution).
   b. Cap the tubes and vortex the GAG solutions.
   c. Dilute the 1 mg/mL GAG standard solutions into labeled microfuge tubes as shown in Table A4.1. Make two independent sets of standards, one from each solution.
   d. Cap the tubes and vortex each standard.

TABLE A4.1
Recipes for Dilution of 1 mg/mL GAG Standard Solution to Generate a Standard Curve

Standard concentration (µg/mL)	125	100	75	50	25	0
GAG standard solution (µL)	125	100	75	50	25	0
TE (µL)	875	900	925	950	975	1000

2. Turn on the plate reader and set the wavelength to A_{525}.

3. Load the standards and samples into a flat-bottom, 96-well plate. As you load the 96-well plate, document in your lab notebook which standard or sample is contained in each well. Do not write on the plate.

   a. Add 40 µL of each standard to a separate well of the 96-well plate.

   b. Vortex each sample and add 40 µL of each sample into separate wells. Repeat so that each sample is measured in duplicate.

   c. Add 360 µL of DMMB dye to each standard and sample.

4. Measure and record A_{525} for each standard and sample. If any sample is out of range of the standards or the spectrophotometer detection limit, dilute the sample more and repeat the measurement until the reading falls within the working range of the calibration curve. Make careful notes in your lab notebook regarding the dilutions.

A4.6 Data Processing and Reporting

The general approach for analyzing data from the DMMB assay is described next. Experiment-specific instructions may also be found in the chapters throughout this text.

1. Enter the absorbance data and GAG concentrations for the standard curve into Excel or a similar program. Plot these data.

   Note: The standards and samples were similarly diluted with the DMMB dye; therefore, the dilution factor can be ignored and the concentration of the samples can be directly compared to that of the standards.

2. The relationship between A_{525} and GAG concentration is nonlinear and can be approximated as a second-order polynomial of the form $y = ax^2 + bx + c$. Fit a second-order polynomial through the standard data and display the coefficients and r^2 value on the plot. The r^2 value describes how strong the relationship is between absorbance and GAG concentration.

3. Using the preceding polynomial equation, determine the concentration and total GAG in each sample.

References

Farndale, R. W., D. J. Buttle, and A. J. Barrett. 1986. Improved quantitation and discrimination of sulphated glycosaminoglycans by use of dimethylmethylene blue. *Biochimica et Biophysica Acta* 883 (2): 173–177.

Farndale, R. W., C. A. Sayers, and A. J. Barrett. 1982. A direct spectrophotometric microassay for sulfated glycosaminoglycans in cartilage cultures. *Connective Tissue Research* 9 (4): 247–248.

Varki, A., R. D. Cummings, J. D. Esko, H. H. Freeze, P. Stanley, C. R. Bertozzi, G. W. Hart, and M. E. Etzler. 2009. *Essentials of glycobiology,* 2nd ed. Cold Spring Harbor, NY: Cold Spring Harbor Laboratory Press.

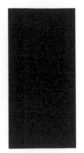

Appendix 5: Microfluidic Device Design and Fabrication

A5.1 Background

Microfluidic technology has application to a wide range of fields, including biological sciences, chemistry, and tissue engineering. Advances in fabrication protocols and the abundance of available designs demonstrate the versatility of this technology. In general, masters are created by "rapid prototyping" involving a combination of high-resolution printing and contact photolithography (Figure A5.1) used to cast replicas in polydimethylsiloxane (PDMS) polymer—specifically, Sylgard® 184 from Dow Corning (Delamarche et al. 1997) (Figure A5.2).

These processes traditionally require use of a clean room/photolithography facility, thereby limiting availability of these protocols in a teaching laboratory environment. However, there is a trend moving the field of microfluidic device fabrication from the clean room to the laboratory bench, eliminating restricting issues such as cost, access, training, and scheduling. This appendix reviews lithographic fabrication techniques associated with clean room access, but in particular highlights several modified techniques for fabrication in the teaching laboratory environment. Several excellent reviews are available to reference these types of protocols (Duffy et al. 1998; McDonald et al. 2000; Rocheleau and Piston 2008).

A5.2 The CAD Drawing

Microdevice fabrication begins with creation of a CAD (computer-aided design) drawing that represents the geometry and actual scaling of the desired device (Figure A5.1). Any computer program that will save designs as encapsulated postscript files (.eps) is appropriate to use (e.g., AutoCAD or Adobe Illustrator). The design should be drawn to scale in black and white. It is easiest to create a black

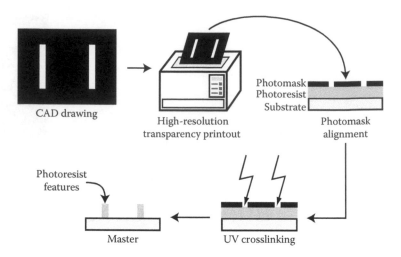

Figure A5.1
Schematic overview of microdevice design and master creation by photolithography. A design of the device features is created to scale as a CAD drawing and printed to film using a high-resolution printer. The printed photomask is aligned to a substrate coated with negative photoresist and exposed regions are cross linked by UV illumination. Non-cross-linked regions are dissolved, leaving a master with photoresist features.

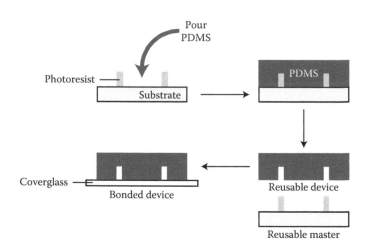

Figure A5.2
Schematic overview of soft lithography. PDMS polymer is poured over the feature side of the master. A cured PDMS mold is then peeled away from the master (which can be reused). If required for fluid flow applications, the PDMS mold can be bonded to a glass slide.

background corresponding to the size of the substrate on which the master will be created and subsequently draw the device specifics to scale in white. If the device requires structures with varied heights, a mask for each height must be generated that can be overlapped using extra design markings during the actual master fabrication process. ***Specialized equipment required:*** CAD software.

A5.3 The Photomask

Depending upon availability of a high-quality printer, a completed CAD drawing may be sent to a professional printer that will print the design to film at high resolution. However, this is not cost effective, particularly if a large number of devices need to be created. Instead, a high-resolution laser printer (>5600 dpi, depending upon the resolution required in the device itself) can be used within the teaching laboratory to print to an acetate transparency (Figure A5.1). Alternative procedures include printing toner to glossy photographic paper (Easley et al. 2009), polyester film (do Lago et al. 2003), or a copper surface (Abdelgawad et al. 2008). Another low-cost alternative involves wax printing (Carrilho, Martinez, and Whitesides 2009). ***Specialized equipment required:*** high-resolution laser printer.

A5.4 Photolithography to Create a Master

Photolithography is the process of using light to transfer geometric shapes (e.g., channels, reservoirs, etc.) from a photomask to the surface of a substrate coated with photoresist, a light-sensitive polymer. There are two types of photoresist: *negative* and *positive*. Positive photoresist exhibits a chemical structure that becomes soluble after exposure to UV light. With a positive photoresist, the photomask protects regions of the photoresist from UV exposure and is an exact replica of the pattern that will remain on the wafer substrate. Conversely, negative photoresist becomes insoluble after exposure to UV light. In this case, the photomask contains the inverse ("negative") pattern of what will remain on the wafer substrate.

It is very important to take this into consideration when determining the black/ white orientation of the CAD design and photomask. Be aware of whether *positive* or *negative* photoresist is required in a protocol. **The following sections briefly describe the main steps involved using SU-8, a negative photoresist, to create a master (Figure A5.1).** SU-8 photoresist is one of the most commonly used reagents in master fabrication; therefore, it is ideal to follow the manufacturer's recommendations (MicroChem, www.microchem.com). ***Specialized equipment required:*** fume hood, digital hot plates, air (or nitrogen) gun, spin coater, UV illuminator, orbital shaker; ***PPE:*** as designated for institution clean room regulations (including bunny suit, hairnet or cap, shoe covers, goggles, and appropriate gloves) or laboratory environment (lab coat, goggles, gloves); ***safety:*** consult MSDS, receive appropriate training, follow proper disposal guidelines.

A5.4.1 Substrate Cleaning

The substrate of choice (e.g., silicon wafer, glass microscope slide) must be thoroughly cleaned prior to use. This will ensure that interfering organic solvents, inorganic contaminants, and particulate matter are removed prior to master fabrication. Clean using either an alcohol series (isopropanol, acetone, isopropanol) or freshly prepared piranha solution (3:1 v/v mixture of sulfuric acid/hydrogen peroxide for 30 minutes). Rinsing in dH_2O is recommended after cleaning. Due to the nature of the cleaning solutions, this step must be done in a fume hood. Solutions should be handled with extreme care and disposed of appropriately.

Safety recommendations: Because piranha solution is highly acidic and a strong oxidizer, it is dangerous and must be handled with extreme care. In the teaching laboratory, it is highly recommended to use the alternative indicated solutions for cleaning purposes. However, if piranha solution is used, a full face shield and rubber gloves should be worn. An acid apron should also be worn over a lab coat. ***Never handle piranha solution unless you have familiarized yourself with MSDSs and relevant standard operating procedures, including proper waste disposal.***

- Dry substrates immediately after cleaning. An air (nitrogen) gun serves this purpose; alternatively, substrates can be placed on a hot plate (65°C for 15 minutes is typically sufficient). The substrates must be clean and dry for optimal processing.
- To ensure that all moisture has been removed from the substrate surface, the sample needs to be surface-baked on a hot plate (200°C for 5 minutes is typically sufficient).

A5.4.2 Photoresist Application

A photoresist (typically SU-8; Microchem Corp.) is spin-coated onto the surface of the cleaned substrate at a desired thickness. It is important to choose photoresist (positive or negative) suited to the photomask. Different resists will result in different thicknesses.

- Gradually heat the substrate using a two-step process (65°C and 95°C) before allowing it to cool.
- Liquid photoresist is spun onto the surface of the substrate. The defined thickness is a function of photoresist viscosity and spin speed. Typically, SU-8 is poured onto the wafer (e.g., 1 mL/SU-8 is required per inch of substrate diameter), which is centered on the spin coater. A vacuum holds the wafer in place while a defined cycling process evenly spreads the photoresist onto the substrate.

A5.4.3 Soft Baking

This step removes/evaporates all solvents from the photoresist and increases the densition of the film. This step may be done on hot plates (or convection oven), and bake times must be optimized for each master. The best results are obtained when temperatures are ramped: low initial temperatures (e.g., 65°C for ~5 minutes) allow solvent to evaporate out of the film at a controlled rate, resulting in better resist–substrate adhesion. This is followed by a higher temperature bake (e.g., 95°C for ~30 minutes). The wafer should then be allowed to cool slowly following a reverse ramp in hot plate temperatures.

A5.4.4 Mask Alignment and UV Exposure

The photomask can now be carefully aligned with the coated substrate for pattern transfer by UV exposure (Figure A5.1). Regions of negative SU-8 photoresist under the clear portions of the photomask are stimulated to polymerize, leaving areas under the dark portions of the mask "protected' (recall that when using a positive resist the opposite will occur and areas under the dark portions of the mask will be "unprotected"). The controlled polymerization/degradation of photoresist when exposed is why the black/white orientation of the CAD drawing is important. *Note: Exposure time to UV illumination is critical and protocol specific; keep in mind that thicker films will require longer exposure.* Due to direct contact between the mask and the photoresist, high-resolution features are possible. However, interfering debris can damage the mask or cause defects in the pattern.

A postexposure bake (also known as a "hard bake") selectively cross links the UV-exposed portions of the film to complete polymerization. This step can be performed on digital hot plates. Bake times should be optimized for each master; however, a two-step bake is recommended (e.g., 65°C and 95°C) to minimize cracking. Similarly, cracking can occur if the master is allowed to cool rapidly.

A5.4.5 Development

Excess unpolymerized photoresist is dissolved away by gentle agitation of the master in SU-8 developer, resulting in a completed master of defined height and geometry (Figure A5.1). While SU-8 developer is optimized for SU-8 photoresist, ethyl lactate and diacetone alcohol can also be used for developing. Thicker films will require increased strength of agitation during development, and the time required (~10 minutes is a good starting point) must be increased with greater thickness.

The master should be rinsed with isopropyl alcohol after development and dried with a gentle stream of air or nitrogen. The appearance of a white film during the rinse step is an indication that the substrate is underdeveloped and should be resubmerged in the developer to repeat the process.

A5.4.6 Hard Baking

A final hard bake is normally not required if SU-8 photoresist has been used during master fabrication. However, this step hardens the photoresist and can increase the smoothness of the desired pattern, particularly if fine structure is a predominant aspect of the desired device. This step also improves adhesion of the photoresist to the substrate surface. A ramped hard bake between 150°C and 200°C on a hot plate will further cross link the material; however, bake times are dependent upon film thickness.

A5.4.7 Storage and Disposal of Masters

Masters should be kept out of direct light and stored in sealed containers, preferably at room temperature. SU-8 masters, if handled carefully, can have a shelf life of ~13 months from the time of fabrication. If broken, masters should be disposed of according to institution regulations for wastes containing similar solvents.

A5.5 PDMS Device Fabrication

Fabrication of a microdevice uses the process of soft lithography, where patterns with features in the nanometer to micrometer range are reproduced using "soft" elastomeric materials such as PDMS. Soft lithography replicates structures defined by a high-relief master (e.g., created in SU-8 negative photoresist by photolithography as described before). PDMS is a highly popular elastomeric substrate for microfluidic fabrication due to easy methods for rapid prototyping. Traditionally, this fabrication occurs within a clean room environment for convenience; however, the low-cost availability of required equipment and careful handling have brought this protocol into the regular laboratory environment. *Specialized equipment required:* top-loading balance, fume hood, digital hot plates, air (or nitrogen) gun, plasma cleaner, vacuum dessicator, curing oven; *PPE:* lab coat, goggles, and gloves; *safety:* consult MSDS and follow proper disposal guidelines

A5.5.1 PDMS Micromolding

The elastomeric polymer PDMS is supplied as a two-part resin that must be thoroughly mixed before pouring over the negative relief master (Figure A5.2). Once cured, the PDMS cast can be removed and used immediately (e.g., as a stamp) or assembled into a device (e.g., microchannels on a microscope slide).

- Use a top-loading balance to measure PDMS as a 10:1 base:cure ratio. This can be mixed thoroughly in a polystyrene petri dish using a combination of stirring and folding (e.g., a plastic fork or hand mixer works well for this purpose). Formation of bubbles is acceptable as it is indicative of a well-stirred emulsion.

- Vacuum desiccation is used to remove the bubbles. Periodic venting and reapplication of the vacuum will accelerate bubble removal from the emulsion.

- Degassed emulsion is poured over the face-up master in a separate polystyrene petri dish. The entire dish can be placed under vacuum to remove any new bubbles introduced during pouring. *Note: Formation of a large bubble beneath the substrate is actually useful as it assists with substrate removal after polymerization.*

- Polymer should be cured at high temperatures (e.g., 95°C for 1 h, 80°C for 2 h, or 70°C for 4 h) using a hot plate or oven. Longer exposure times are required if using lower curing temperatures (which can eliminate the need for hot plates).

- Cured polymer should be carefully removed from the petri dish using a thin spatula. Care must be taken not to break or damage the relatively inflexible master. "Edge and peel" as you work your way around the dish.

- Excess PDMS should be cut away from under the master.

- The PDMS cast can be placed feature-side up on a clean, nontreated petri dish to cut out individual devices. Gloves must be worn to prevent deposition of skin oils or fingerprints onto the cast.

- Devices created for micropatterning protocols can be stored in a clean petri dish prior to use.

- Other devices may require functional details such as portholes for use as tube access or on-chip reservoirs. A #3 cork borer with a beveled edge is recommended for large reservoirs. For tube access ports, a needle hole is made that is slightly smaller than the outer diameter of the tubing being used, to ensure adequate sealing to fluidic pressures. A blunt 18-gauge needle that exhibits a beveled edge by repeated insertion of a thin wire is an ideal starting point, although trouble-shooting will be required to optimize.

A5.5.2 PDMS-Substrate Bonding

Microdevices created with channels or reservoirs for observation of fluid flow require bonding to a substrate, such as a glass microscope slide or coverslip, for experimental and observation purposes (Figure A5.2). If samples require fluorescence microscopy, it is ideal to use thin glass coverslips rather than microscope slides for better working distance with high-resolution objectives.

- It is extremely important to be certain that both the PDMS cast and substrate are cleaned and dried prior to bonding. Clear adhesive tape can be used to clear working surfaces of dust and polymer fragments. Place clean tape against surface and gently pull away; debris will adhere to the tape and be removed.

- The substrate should be cleaned of organic residues using methanol and acetone, acetone and isopropanol, or piranha solution (as described in Section A5.4.1). Substrates should be fully dried using an air or nitrogen gun.

- The PDMS cast can be irreversibly bonded to the clean substrate via oxygen plasma treatment. Both cast and substrate are briefly surface treated using plasma cleaner treatment (e.g., Harrick Plasma, Ithaca, NY). The duration can range from 30 s to several minutes, depending on the instrumentation used. Remember that the PDMS cast should be treated directly on the features side.

- *Immediately* use forceps or tweezers to place the PDMS cast carefully feature-side down onto the treated substrate. Some bubbles may appear, but they will disappear with time. A spatula can be used to press down on the PDMS to assist in bonding to the glass slide: slowly guide from one side to the other.

- The device can also be placed on a 70°C hot plate for 5–30 minutes to ensure that covalent bonding occurs. Gently squeeze the PDMS to determine if it has bonded; it should not detach from the glass surface with any degree of pressure.

- Once polyethylene tubing has been inserted into the appropriate ports of the assembled devices, 5 minutes epoxy can be used to secure them in place. Ensure that epoxy is placed completely around each tube where it meets the PDMS mold as it also serves as a seal. Allow to cure overnight.

- A second seal can be created by completely covering the epoxy with 100% clear silicone rubber sealant. This protects the epoxy seals, which may break easily and cause the devices to leak. Allow to dry overnight before use.

A5.5.3 Storage and Disposal of PDMS Devices

If devices have been prepared in advance, they can be stored by stacking between aluminum foil, which prevents irreversible bonding between devices. Devices should be handled carefully to prevent breaking or separation from the bonded substrate. Prepolymerized PDMS is messy and will stick to surfaces. The mixing area will become coated with PDMS. Placing lab-bench paper in the mixing area is recommended. Any spills that occur will be easiest to clean up if the PDMS is left to cure, as the solid polymer can be scraped away. Dispose of used or broken devices according to institution regulations for waste containing similar polymers.

A5.6 Teaching Laboratory Alternatives

The ability to experience master fabrication in a teaching environment is often impeded by equipment cost, time requirements associated with the protocols, and required access to a clean room/photolithography facility. However, if a clean work area is available, including a designated fume hood, it is possible to establish the master fabrication protocol in the teaching laboratory. Appropriate PPE should always be worn, not only to protect oneself but also to keep masters and devices as clean as possible during fabrication. ***Recommendations for master fabrication small equipment purchase:*** digital hot plates (Chemat digital hot plates, programmable, Sigma #Z551597, ~$2,900 each), orbital shaker (Belly Dancer Agitator, Fisher Scientific #15-453-211 ~$1,800), nitrogen gun (Entegris, #421-42-11, ~$140), spin coater (MTI Corporation, programmable compact spin coater—500–8000 rpm, 4 ft wafer max + accessories—~$2,800), UV illumination source (handheld long wavelength—365 nm—UV lamp, Spectroline ENF-240C, Fisher Scientific, ~$250).

Should a laboratory budget not allow for purchase of equipment required for traditional photolithography protocols, advances in fabrication technology are making alternative (and appealing) strategies available. However, when navigating away from traditional protocols, one must keep in mind biomaterial incompatibility as well as other considerations such as the limitations of feature resolution. Many of these alternatives are suitable for teaching-laboratory environments and provide intriguing options to standard fabrication protocols.

A5.6.1 Producing the Photomask

Professional print shops were once commonly used to create photomask films, but this task is now commonly performed in house in laboratories by using high-resolution laser printers. The CAD drawing is typically printed at high resolution to an acetate transparency (Fisher Scientific is one supplier). However, diverging protocols make use of other print platforms, such as photo paper (Easley et al. 2009) or copper films (Abdelgawad et al. 2008).

A5.6.2 Alternate UV Sources

Several recent studies provide intriguing options for the UV cross-linking step of photolithography and may be suitable for teaching laboratory protocols, depending upon the UV energy requirements. A handheld, long wavelength (365 nm) UV lamp (Spectroline ENF-240C, Fisher Scientific) was successfully used to demonstrate photopolymerization of a prepolymer photoresist solution (Berkowski et al. 2005). The light generated by a laminar cell culture BSC has also been used to fabricate poly(ethylene glycol) diacrylate (PEGDA) microstructures successfully by photolithography (Hwang et al. 2010). This is an attractive option since teaching laboratories are commonly outfitted with culture hoods. Finally, the low cost and compact format make a solid-state photolithography (SSP) system constructed from an array of UV light-emitting diodes (LEDs) an appealing instrument for a teaching laboratory (Huntington and Odom 2011). Powered by regular "AA" batteries, this illumination source is capable of creating photoresist patterns with critical features ~ 200 nm across 4 in. silicon wafers without requiring a vacuum source or clean room facility.

A5.6.3 Master Creation without Photolithography

Of greater relevance to teaching laboratories is the opportunity to create masters without the restrictions of using a clean room/photolithography facility. Several (but certainly not all) interesting options are described in this section.

- **Toner transfer masking** is an in-lab protocol using commercially available thin brass strips as a substrate for master fabrication (Easley et al. 2009). CAD drawings are printed to glossy photo paper using a single toner laser printer (e.g., HP LaserJet 4350n; 1200 dpi). The toner is printed to the starch layer of this photomask alternative. A regular clothing iron is used at the highest setting to transfer the ink from the paper to the brass strip (e.g., 0.813 mm; 10 minutes transfer). The paper is peeled away after soaking in room-temperature water (10 minutes). The non-inked brass is etched at a defined rate and depth using an ammonium persulfate solution (20% w/v), leaving a photomask that has been created in a period of time suited to a laboratory session. This protocol also avoids clean room requirements and is a low-cost alternative to photolithography.

- **Copper "masters on demand"** are another alternative for quick fabrication of masters in the laboratory without photolithography (Abdelgawad et al. 2008). In this case, a Xerox Phaser 6360N color printer was used to transfer CAD patterns to flexible copper-coated films (DuPont Electronic Materials). The films were consequently immersed in CE-100 copper etchant (Transene Company Inc; 60°C; <10 minutes) until exposed copper was etched away. Dicing tape (Semiconductor Equipment Corporation) was used to protect the non-inked copper back side. On some occasions, multiple layers of toner were required to resist etching; however, the resulting masters were found to be robust and of appropriate resolution to create channels as narrow as 100 μm and with depths of 9–70 μm. Due to the short fabrication time frame and nonrequirement for a photolithography facility, this technique is also appropriate for a teaching-laboratory environment.

- **"Shrinky dinks"** is an interesting fabrication protocol that makes use of the commercially available children's craft product (www.shrinkydinks.com). The protocol is based on the principle that these thermoplastic sheets reduce their size when heated above transition temperatures. The CAD design is printed directly to a sheet that is shrunk to become the master (Grimes et al. 2008). Following standard soft lithography protocols, PDMS polymer is poured directly onto the "shrink dink" master to create a mold. This study demonstrated a minimum line width of 65 μm and achieved multiple feature heights by reprinting the channels. Likewise, this technique has a short time requirement, does not require spin-coating or UV cross-linking, and can be studied in a teaching-laboratory environment.

- **Wax printing** protocols make use of consumer-grade wax printers (i.e., printers that print with a wax-based ink) to form the desired features of the master (Carrilho et al. 2009; Kaigala et al. 2007). For example, Kaigala et al. used a Xerox Phaser 8500DN printer at its highest resolution setting (2400 FinePoint2) to print designs to photo film (Mylar, Fuji Photo Film Canada Inc.) or transparency film (Phaser solid ink professional transparency film). Both substrates were found to exhibit excellent adhesion to wax, resulting in sharp features as compared to laser printer output. The printed transparency serves as the master for traditional PDMS-based soft lithography. The polymer is cured at room temperature, thereby removing the requirement for heat sources. Although some variations in channel width were detected, a maximum height of 10 μm could be achieved. This technique is also suitable for testing in a teaching laboratory as it can be performed (master fabrication and device creation) within several hours.

- **Nylon mesh** is an intriguing alternative to PDMS-casted stamping for micropatterning extracellular matrices in cell culture assays (Zawko and Schmidt 2010). This particular protocol avoids not only the use of direct printing, photolithography, and soft lithography, but also the requirements to work in a clean room facility. Nylon 6/6 screening mesh (Small Parts Inc.) was dipped into hydrogel solutions (e.g., 1%, w/v, aqueous alginate; chitosan) and placed onto treated glass slides or tissue-culture polystyrene substrates. The samples were air-dried at room temperature (thereby removing the requirement for a heat source) and dipped into liquid nitrogen (10 s). Once the mesh was removed, a hydrogel grid remained on the culture surface that was dessicated and cross linked (2 minutes). Therefore, in a very short period of time and with minimum equipment requirements, matrix grids were prepared and available for cell seeding experiments. This commercially available mesh can be purchased with various sizes of open squares for controlling pattern size and comparing culture density effects.

References

Abdelgawad, M., M. W. Watson, E. W. Young, J. M. Mudrik, M. D. Ungrin, and A. R. Wheeler. 2008. Soft lithography: Masters on demand. *Lab Chip* 8 (8): 1379–1385.

Berkowski, K. L., K. N. Plunkett, Q. Yu, and J. S. Moore. 2005. Introduction to photolithography: Preparation of microscale polymer silhouettes. *Journal of Chemical Education* 82 (9): 1365–1369.

Carrilho, E., A. W. Martinez, and G. M. Whitesides. 2009. Understanding wax printing: A simple micropatterning process for paper-based microfluidics. *Analytical Chemistry* 81 (16): 7091–7095.

Delamarche, E., H. Schmid, B. Michel, and H. Biebuyck. 1997. Stability of molded polydimethylsiloxane microstructures. *Advanced Materials* 9 (9): 741–746.

do Lago, C. L., H. D. da Silva, C. A. Neves, J. G. Brito-Neto, and J. A. da Silva. 2003. A dry process for production of microfluidic devices based on the lamination of laser-printed polyester films. *Analytical Chemistry* 75 (15): 3853–3858.

Duffy, D. C., J. C. McDonald, O. J. Schueller, and G. M. Whitesides. 1998. Rapid prototyping of microfluidic systems in poly(dimethylsiloxane). *Analytical Chemistry* 70 (23): 4974–4984.

Easley, C. J., R. K. Benninger, J. H. Shaver, W. Steven Head, and D. W. Piston. 2009. Rapid and inexpensive fabrication of polymeric microfluidic devices via toner transfer masking. *Lab Chip* 9 (8): 1119–1127.

Grimes, A., D. N. Breslauer, M. Long, J. Pegan, L. P. Lee, and M. Khine. 2008. Shrinky–Dink microfluidics: Rapid generation of deep and rounded patterns. *Lab Chip* 8 (1): 170–172.

Huntington, M. D., and T. W. Odom. 2011. A portable, benchtop photolithography system based on a solid-state light source. *Small* 7 (22): 3144–3147.

Hwang, C. M., W. Y. Sim, S. H. Lee, A. M. Foudeh, H. Bae, and A. Khademhosseini. 2010. Benchtop fabrication of PDMS microstructures by an unconventional photolithographic method. *Biofabrication* 2 (4): 045001.

Kaigala, G. V., S. Ho, R. Penterman, and C. J. Backhouse. 2007. Rapid prototyping of microfluidic devices with a wax printer. *Lab Chip* 7 (3): 384–387.

McDonald, J. C., D. C. Duffy, J. R. Anderson, D. T. Chiu, H. Wu, O. J. Schueller, and G. M. Whitesides. 2000. Fabrication of microfluidic systems in poly(dimethylsiloxane). *Electrophoresis* 21 (1): 27–40.

Rocheleau, J. V., and D. W. Piston. 2008. Chapter 4: Combining microfluidics and quantitative fluorescence microscopy to examine pancreatic islet molecular physiology. *Methods in Cell Biology* 89:71–92.

Zawko, S. A., and C. E. Schmidt. 2010. Simple benchtop patterning of hydrogel grids for living cell microarrays. *Lab Chip* 10 (3): 379–383.

Index

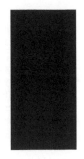

E

Early passage cell line, 53
ECM islands, 109
Effective viscosity, 199
    and capillary radius, 201
    as function of microchannel width, 201
    and velocity in microchannel, 200
    and vessel size, 197
Elastic cartilage, 41
Elastic modulus
    of cells, 207
    half-space model, 208
Electronic balance, 2
    cleaning, 18
    lab skills, 17–18
    leveling, 18
    range, 17
    weighing powder sample, 18
Embryonic development, laminin role in, 92
Emergency contact numbers, 10
Emergency procedures, 12
Emergency showers, 9
Emission spectra, PicoGreen DNA-binding dye, 246
Engineering controls, 9–10
Enzymatic decellularization methods, 80
Enzyme activity per volume, 48
Enzyme concentration, 48
Equipment
    bone material properties experiment, 222
    cell counting, 242
    cell patterning, 113
    cell population growth modeling, 59
    cell population motility, 128
    cell population purification, 73
    cell seeding onto biomaterial scaffolds, 103
    citing manufacturers, 229
    collagen gel contraction, 139
    decellularized matrices, 82
    DMMB assay, 250
    Fahraeus-Lindqvist effect experiment, 203
    matrix accumulation experiment, 164
    microcontact printing (μCP), 113
    microfluidic micropipette aspiration, 212
    PicoGreen DNA assay, 246
    plating density and cell adhesion, 94
    shared, xvi
    stem cell fate experiment, 181–182
    substrate stiffness experiment, 150
Equipment operation, 17
Erlenmeyer flasks, 2
Error bars, 141
EthD-1, pork tenderloin stained with, 84

Ethidium homodimer (EthD-1) probe, 43
EtOH rinses, 88
Excitation spectra, PicoGreen DNA-binding dye, 246
Experiment overview
    bone material properties, 220
    cell patterning, 111–112
    cell population growth, 57
    cell population motility, 128
    cell population purification, 70–71
    cell seeding onto biomaterial scaffolds, 102
    collagen gel contraction, 137
    decellularized matrices, 80–81
    Fahraeus-Lindqvist effect, 201–202
    matrix accumulation, 163
    microcontact printing (μCP), 111–112
    microfluidic micropipette aspiration, 211–212
    plating density and cell adhesion, 93
    stem cell fate experiment, 179–180
    substrate stiffness and cell differentiation, 148–149
Experimental findings, xvi, 227
Experimental results
    reporting as text, 230–231
    reporting in figures, 231–232
    reporting in tables, 231
Exponential growth, 54, 55, 95
Exponential growth equation, 55–56
Extended abstracts, 227, 233–234
Extracellular matrix (ECM), 41, 79, 91
    in articular cartilage, 161
    collagens, multiadhesive matrix proteins, and proteoglycans in, 91
    design criteria for artificial, 92
    injectable form of decellularized, 79
    material properties, 145
    remodeling processes, 135
    role in stem cell fate decisions, 174
    structural proteins remaining in, 88
Eyewash, 9
EZ-Link-Sulfo-NHS-LC-Biotin, 71, 73

F

Face shields, 10, 11
Fahraeus-Lindqvist effect, 197–200
    cell velocity measurement through microchannels, 203–205
    data processing, 205
    equipment and supplies, 203
    experimental setup, 204
    learning objectives, 200–201
    materials, 203
    methods, 203–205

O

Objective, choosing correct, 25–26
Objective lens, changing, 26–27
Objective statements
  in extended abstracts, 233
  in technical reports, 229
Occupational Safety and Health Administration
  (OSHA), 11
Oil immersion lenses, 26
One-way ANOVA, 98, 142
Online references, 232
Orbital shaker, 2, 3, 255, 260
Organic solvent, pipetting for liquid transfer, 19
Organogenesis, 137
Osmolarity, effects on ECM synthesis, 171
Osteoarthritis, 161
Osteogenesis imperfecta (OI), 218, 225
Osteoimplants, 220
Osteoporosis, 217, 225

P

p-values, 230
PA hydrogel stiffness, 145
  fluorescent microsphere measurement
    method, 146
  measurement methods, 146
  microball method, 146
PA hydrogels
  advantages, 145
  calculating using microscope technique, 154
  cell seeding onto functionalized, 153–154
  characterizing dimensions and material
    properties, 155–156
  cross-link density, 158
  fabrication, 148
  functionalizing with Type I collagen, 152–153
  maximum possible density, 158
  preparation, 151–152
  recipes for varying stiffness, 152
  resistance to passive protein absorption, 148
  suggested format for gel deformation data,
    157
Parabolic velocity, in rectangular microchannel,
  200
Paracrine capture probabilities, 177
Paracrine signaling, 174, 176
  stochastic model, 183–185
Particle streak velocity images, 201
Passaging cell cultures, 34–36, 53, 64, 65
Pasteur pipettes, 7, 15, 31
  for liquid transfer, 22–23
Pathogenic processes, ECM remodeling in, 135

Patterned cells, imaging, 116–117
PBE, 59, 103, 165, 250
PBS, 98
PBS + P/113S
PDMS, 109
PDMS device fabrication, 258
  device storage and disposal, 260
  micro molding, 258–259
  substrate bonding, 259–260
PDMS micromolding, 258–259
PDMS polymer, 253
PDMS stamps, 111, 201, 254
  fabrication for engineering stem cell fate, 175,
    179, 190
  master fabrication, 188–189
  in microchannel devices, 202
PDMS-substrate bonding, 259–260
Peak strain, 225
Peer-reviewed journal articles, 228
Penicillin and streptomycin (P/S) additive, 30
Percent viability, cell suspension, 38
Percentiles, 230
Personal protective equipment, 10–11, 93, 255,
  258
Personnel safety, 9
pH meter, 3
Phase contrast, 6
Phase slider adjustment, 26
Phenotype-specific behaviors, loss with
  culturing, 53
Phosphate-buffered saline (PBS), 81
Photolithography, 201, 202. *See also* Soft
  lithography
  to create master, 255
Photomask, 255
  production, 261
Photoresist application, 256
Physical characteristics, 11
Physical decellularization methods, 79–80
Physical hazards, 11
PicoGreen, 59, 80, 102, 104, 162, 165, 246
  DNA assay with, 245–248
  as potential mutagen, 58
PicoGreen assay, 54, 62–63
  mutagenicity and toxicity, 57
  sample collection for, 61
PicoGreen DNA-binding dye, emission and
  excitation spectra, 246
Pipette aids, 3, 18
  for liquid transfer, 18–19
Pipette tips, 7
Pipettes
  barrier tips, 22
  cross-contamination issues, 22

Milton Keynes UK
Ingram Content Group UK Ltd.
UKHW031144141024
449569UK00024B/1072